Managing Obesity

A Clinical Guide

Gary D. Foster, PhD, and Cathy A. Nonas, MS, RD, CDE
Editors

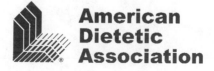

American Dietetic Association

Diana Faulhaber, Publisher
Jason M. Muzinic, Acquisitions Editor
Elizabeth Nishiura, Production Editor

The views expressed in this publication are those of the authors and do not necessarily reflect policies and/or official positions of the American Dietetic Association. Mention of product names in this publication does not constitute endorsement by the authors or the American Dietetic Association. The American Dietetic Association disclaims responsibility for the application of the information contained herein.

10 9 8 7 6 5 4 3 2

Library of Congress Cataloging-in-Publication Data

Managing obesity : a clinical guide / Gary D. Foster and Cathy A. Nonas, editors.
   p. ; cm.
Includes bibliographical references and index.
  ISBN 0-88091-334-7
  1. Obesity—Treatment.
  [DNLM: 1. Obesity—therapy. 2. Health Behavior. 3. Patient
Education. WD 210 M2673 2003] I. Foster, Gary D., 1959– II. Nonas,
Cathy.

  RC628.M348 2003
  616.3'9806—dc22

                                               2003015314

To my mother, Jean, and late father, Don, with love and gratitude
—Gary D. Foster

To my children, Sasha, Aurora, and Lucy
—Cathy A. Nonas

Contents

Contributors

Louis J. Aronne, MD
Weill-Cornell Medical College
New York, NY

Steven N. Blair, PED
The Cooper Institute
Dallas, TX

Mary Pat Bolton, MA, RD
Medical Writer
Houston, TX

Ruth Ann Carpenter, MS, RD
The Cooper Institute
Dallas, TX

Patricia S. Choban MD
Department of Human Nutrition
The Ohio State University
Columbus, OH

Gary D. Foster, PhD
University of Pennsylvania School
   of Medicine
Philadelphia, PA

Molly Gee, MEd, RD
Baylor Medical Center
Houston, TX

Holly Herzog, MS, RD
University of Nevada School of
   Medicine
Reno, NV

Eileen Kennedy, DSc, RD
Columbia University, Mailman
   School of Public Health
New York, NY

Betty Kovacs, MS, RD
St. Luke's-Roosevelt Hospital
New York, NY

Doina Kulick, MD
University of Nevada School of
   Medicine
Reno, NV

Angie Makris, PhD, RD
University of Pennsylvania School
   of Medicine
Philadelphia, PA

Allison Schimmel Matson, MS, RD
Private Practice Consultant
Yardley, PA

Cathy A. Nonas, MS, RD, CDE
North General Hospital
New York, NY

Suzanne Phelan, PhD
The Miriam Hospital
Brown Medical School
Providence, RI

F. Xavier Pi-Sunyer, MD, MPH
New York Obesity Research Center
New York, NY

Rebecca Reeves, PhD, RD
Baylor College of Medicine
Houston, TX

Siri Sirichanvimol, MS, RD
New York University Medical Center
New York, NY

Sachiko T. St. Jeor, PhD, RD
University of Nevada School of
    Medicine
Reno, NV

Bonnie Taub-Dix, MA, RD, CDN
Private Practice Consultant
New York, NY

Thomas A. Wadden, PhD
University of Pennsylvania School
    of Medicine
Philadelphia, PA

Jonathan A. Waitman, MD
Weill-Cornell Medical College
New York, NY

Rena R. Wing, PhD
Brown Medical School
Providence, RI

Reviewers

Olivia Kelly, RD, CNSD
St. Vincent's Catholic Medical
  Center
New York, NY

Alice K. Lindeman, PhD, RD
Associate Professor
Indiana University
Bloomington, IN

Louise W. Peck, PhD, RD
Clinical Nutrition Manager
St. Joseph Medical Center
Tacoma, WA

Helen M. Seagle, MS, RD
Program Director
Weight Management Program
Kaiser Permanente, CO

Laurie Tansman, MS, RD, CDN
Nutrition Coordinator
Mt. Sinai Hospital
New York, NY

Acknowledgments

We would like to thank each of the contributors for crafting state-of-the-art accounts about the research and treatment of obesity. Their willingness and enthusiasm to help write a clinically based book on obesity were central to this undertaking.

From the American Dietetic Association, we would like to thank Jason Muzinic, acquisitions editor, for shepherding this book from its earliest stages, and Elizabeth Nishiura, production editor, for her production expertise—this book is on time because of them. We are also very grateful to Christine Reidy, executive director, Commission on Dietetic Registration, for having the vision to start a Weight Management Certificate Course. It was that course and its faculty that gave us the idea for this book.

We would like to acknowledge all of our patients who have shared their struggles about weight management, and taught us so much over the years. They are the reason for this book. Likewise, we thank each of our colleagues who continue in the battle to treat overweight and obesity more effectively. This book incorporates many of their teachings.

I (GDF) would like thank my wife, Kathleen, for her love and support and my children, Katie, Ryan, and Kevin, for teaching me that work is not all that important.

I (CAN) would like to thank Ted VanItallie, MD, for help on my chapters. His wisdom is always inspiring. Thank you to Mark Smith for helping edit some pretty tough paragraphs and to Shirley Person for reading chapters as they flew out of her copy machine. Finally, thanks go to my children, Sasha, Aurora, and Lucy, for bearing with me when the "closet was too full."

—Gary D. Foster and Cathy A. Nonas, editors

Foreword

Preparing dietetics professionals to compete and be knowledgeable in the emerging area of food and nutrition is the foundation of the American Dietetic Association's (ADA's) strategic plan. ADA recognizes that obesity in the United States is reaching epidemic proportions, and that we, as dietetics professionals, must be ready to address the multifaceted issues surrounding this public health problem.

This publication, *Managing Obesity: A Clinical Guide,* provides dietitians and other health care professionals with the current research on obesity and weight management as well as practical guidelines for using that information. The distinguished list of contributors to this book exemplifies the philosophy that a multidisciplinary team is important in establishing a successful weight program for our clients. The editors, Gary D. Foster, PhD, and Cathy A. Nonas, MS, RD, CDE, direct the practitioner through the obesity maze with the assistance of experts in the various aspects of weight management. From assessment and clinical management to behavioral treatment and dietary approaches, this book places the latest research and practical applications at the practitioner's fingertips. Physical activity as a key component of weight loss and weight management is highlighted in this book, with contributors providing insights into the ways dietetics professionals can help clients become more physically active. Numerous case studies are provided to illustrate methods of intervention. The sections on pharmacological and surgical treatments provide guidelines for helping clients to evaluate whether various interventions will meet their individualized needs.

A weight management program is successful when a health care practitioner truly assesses an individual's health status, behavioral change pattern, and physical activity ability. Developing an individualized approach to weight management is the underlying theme in this "must have" reference.

My thanks to Gary Foster and Cathy Nonas for their work on this timely book. *Managing Obesity: A Clinical Guide* provides dietetics professionals and all other health care practitioners with the knowledge to address an escalating public health problem in the United States—obesity.

Marianne Smith Edge, MS, RD, FADA
President
American Dietetic Association

Introduction

Why Another Book On Obesity?

There are several excellent books on the complex topic of obesity. Typically, these works have a strong research focus with less emphasis on the practical aspects of clinical care. In contrast, this book is meant primarily for clinicians. Dietitians are on the frontlines of the obesity epidemic, but many others (including exercise specialists, physical therapists, nurses, nurse practitioners, psychologists, and social workers) are helping individuals manage their eating and activity in a healthful manner. Although we expect that physicians will find this book useful, this book was written principally for nonphysicians and includes a chapter on teaming with physicians for effective clinical monitoring. Very few physicians have the time in a brief office visit to treat obesity comprehensively, and obesity cannot be confined to any one discipline. It will take physicians and nonphysicians alike to reinforce the message that modest weight loss can have significant health benefits. Therefore, this book has been written to help all clinicians to understand and treat overweight and obesity better and to stem the tide of further medical complications.

Structure of Managing Obesity

Although prevention is the best way to confront the obesity epidemic, clinicians must still face the challenge one patient at a time. How clinicians face this challenge will depend on the kind of office they work in and their specialty, as well as the needs of the patient. However, having an appreciation of the complexity of the problem and the numerous treatment options

1

available can enhance any perspective. We hope that this book provides clinicians on the frontlines with a broad range of options to help treat their patients effectively. Topics include assessment, medical monitoring, diets, pharmacotherapy, surgery, physical activity, behavior modification, and maintenance of weight loss.

Chapters are typically divided into two parts: Part A, an Overview section that reviews current research and treatment guidelines and, Part B, a Practical Applications section that translates guidelines into practice. The Overview sections have been written by some of the most renowned experts in their fields. These chapters are concise and authoritative accounts of the science behind clinical guidelines. They are helpful in identifying what is known and what is yet to be learned in this burgeoning field of obesity research as it relates to clinical care.

The Practical Applications sections are authored by seasoned clinicians, most of whom are also clinical researchers. These sections provide guidance on what to do and how to do it, and they consider whether guidelines need to be adjusted in order to meet the constraints of normal clinical practice. Numerous case studies illustrate the principles and approaches discussed in the chapters.

Nomenclature

In many of the chapters, the words "overweight" and "obesity" are used interchangeably, even though the two terms are not technically synonyms (see Chapter 1: Obesity: An Overview). Many of the topics covered in this book, such as weight loss maintenance, physical activity, behavior, and diet, address issues that are important to both obesity and overweight, so in these contexts it is not crucial to distinguish between the two categories. In other chapters, such as Chapter 7: Pharmacological Treatment and Chapter 8: Surgical Treatment, body mass index criteria are specifically delineated.

The words "client" and "patient" are also used interchangeably, since clinicians use both and usually favor one over the other. There are cases to be made for each term. In specific clinical situations (eg, inpatient settings), one term may make more sense. In general, however, both terms are used throughout this book.

Using This Book

There are at least two ways to use this book. The first is as a guide to effective clinical skills in the treatment of obesity. Whether you see the patient in a private office or a hospital setting, the information in the Practical Applications sections will help you assess and treat the patient/client more holistically, looking at the gamut of environmental, cultural, and medical issues that affect the obese person. Second, this book can help practitioners determine when it is appropriate to refer an individual to other professionals. For example, the psychologist may not need to know how to monitor a patient's vital signs during weight loss, but it is imperative that the patient who is losing (or gaining) weight be referred back to the primary care physician for follow-up evaluation. Who better to remind the patient of this than the practitioner the patient is seeing on a regular basis?

The Challenge

Treating obesity is exciting, frustrating, inspiring, and draining—sometimes all in the same day. There will be days when you question your professional skills and competence. On those days, remember that obesity is a chronic, refractory condition that requires chronic care of varying intensities. Also, although it will likely not be cured in the near future, there are encouraging signs that obesity will be managed more efficiently as more medications, currently in research, are introduced. There is no doubt that weight control is tough work, and that it takes tremendous effort to defend against an environment that prompts individuals to eat more and move less. But the effort required to meet this challenge is more than worth it. To that end, it is important to remind ourselves, and our patients, that small weight losses bring big improvements in health and quality of life. As we have learned from the National Weight Control Registry, people can lose weight and keep it off! This book offers the clinician methods for helping overweight and obese patients do just that.

Chapter 1

Obesity: An Overview

Cathy A. Nonas, MS, RD, CDE, and Gary D. Foster, PhD

Obesity is so pervasive in modern society that clinicians of all types and specialties address this issue on a daily basis. As a result, the need to better understand and to treat obesity is essential in effective clinical practice. This introductory chapter provides an overview of the problem of obesity—its consequences, assessment, etiology, and treatments.

The Problem of Obesity

Consequences

The rationale for treating obesity seriously lies in its adverse medical consequences. Adults who are overweight (body mass index [BMI] ≥ 25, 65 inches, 150 lb) or obese (BMI ≥ 30, 65 inches, 180 lb) are at increased risk for early mortality (1,2), as well as for a variety of medical conditions that include type 2 diabetes, hypertension, dyslipidemia, cardiovascular disease, and sleep apnea (3,4). Recent data suggest that obesity accounts for 14% to 20% of all cancer deaths, making it second only to smoking in terms of modifiable risk factors for cancer mortality (2). Obesity also has significant economic costs, approaching $117 billion annually in the United States (4). The psychosocial consequences of obesity include body image disparagement, impaired quality of life, and, among the severely obese, depression (5,6).

The seriousness of obesity is exacerbated by its increasing prevalence. A recent analysis from the Centers for Disease Control and Prevention (CDC) indicates that 34% of Americans are overweight and 31% are obese (7). Thus, 65% of the nation has a BMI ≥ 25, compared with 56% in 1994 and 46% in 1980 (7,8). The number of obese Americans has more than doubled (15% to 31%) during the last 20 years (7,8), and the number of severely obese persons (BMI ≥ 40) has nearly tripled in the last decade (9). It is estimated that, at this rate, the entire adult population will be overweight or obese by 2030 (10). American children are following in the footsteps of American adults: obesity among US children is increasing at a rate of 20% to 30% per decade (11). The medical costs alone to maintain this population will be prohibitive. The serious nature and increasing prevalence of obesity have prompted calls for action from the World Health Organization (WHO) (12) and from the US Surgeon General (13).

With all this bad news, it is heartening to realize that small weight losses (5% to 10%) are associated with significant improvements in health outcomes such as glycemic control, dyslipidemia, and hypertension, among others (3). These improvements, as well as the reductions in waist circumference that accompany weight loss, have positive effects on the metabolic syndrome and other risk factors.

Assessment

Formerly, relative weight was assessed as percent of ideal body weight (based on height and gender), using life insurance actuarial tables (14). The ideal weights, however, were flawed in several ways (eg, an overrepresentation of males and those of high enough socioeconomic status to purchase life insurance) (15). Moreover, the outcome of interest was mortality, so the risk of morbidity could not be assessed. During the last decade, BMI has supplanted percent of ideal weight as the preferred method to document relative weight in patient charts. BMI is calculated as weight in kg/ht in m^2. It is most easily assessed with height and weight grids (16) or by the following formula:

1. Multiply weight in pounds by 703 = A
2. Divide A by height in inches = B
3. Divide B by height in inches = BMI

Although it is best to measure both height and weight, clinicians who do not have scales in their offices, such as psychologists and social workers, can assess BMI using patient estimates.

Table 1.1 presents the various National Heart, Lung, and Blood Institute (NHLBI) and WHO categories, based on BMI. In general, the higher the

Table 1.1.   Weight Classifications Based on BMI

Category	BMI
Underweight	< 18.5
Normal	18.5–24.9
Overweight	25.0–29.9
Class I obesity	30.0–34.9
Class II obesity	35.0–39.9
Class III obesity (Extreme obesity)	≥ 40

Data are from references 3 and 12.

BMI, the higher the risk of morbidity and mortality (see Chapter 3: Clinical Monitoring). Before 1998, the United States used the criterion of BMI > 27 for overweight. In 1998, the National Institutes of Health lowered the criterion to match the WHO's guidelines for overweight as BMI ≥ 25 (3). Some have considered this homage to a thinner ideal; it is not. The shift to a lower BMI mirrors the same philosophy that the American Diabetes Association displayed with its recent shift to a lower blood glucose as the sign of frank diabetes. The concern was that too many people were undiagnosed, and that a lower criterion for diabetes would spur clinicians into action sooner. This was the same rationale for lowering the criterion for overweight: that more "at risk" people would be treated earlier, thereby reducing concomitant health problems inherent in this susceptible subset of the population.

Risk is also affected by the amount of intra-abdominal fat. Several large epidemiological studies have demonstrated that, independent of BMI, abdominal fat distribution is associated with a greater risk for ischemic heart disease, hypertension, stroke, and mortality (17,18). Waist circumference serves as good clinical proxy for computed tomography (CT) and magnetic resonance imaging (MRI) assessments of intra-abdominal adipose tissue. An upper-body fat distribution is defined as a waist circumference ≥ 35 inches for women and ≥ 40 inches for men. Among patients with a BMI ≥ 35, measuring waist circumference is not indicated, since the risk due to BMI alone is already very significant. Waist circumference is best measured around the abdomen at the level of the iliac crest (16) (see Chapter 2: Assessment).

Therefore, it is not good clinical practice to leave untreated a woman with a BMI of 26, a waist circumference of 37 inches, and a family history of type 2 diabetes. Treatment may include prevention of further weight gain, adoption of healthier lifestyle behaviors, and/or referral to an appropriate specialist. If the health care professional does not make the connection between this woman's weight, waist circumference, lifestyle, personal history, and family history, then her risk of converting to type 2 diabetes in the near future is greater. If the clinician can make the appropriate connection, and the woman can become educated about physical activity and nutrition—and stop further weight gain—then the patient may indeed prevent or at least delay the onset of diabetes. To make the appropriate connections about health and patient care, BMI and waist circumference become vital statistics, and any chart is incomplete without reference to them.

Office Environment

Every office, no matter what kind, should be sensitive to the different needs of obese patients (see Chapter 4: Behavioral Treatment). If nothing else, there should be at least one sturdy chair without arms for those with extra-wide girth and weights of > 300 pounds. If part of the monitoring process is measuring weight, then the scale should be able to measure >350 pounds, have a wide platform that is low to the ground for the patient to step on, and a support bar for the patient to grab hold of. Individuals who measure waist circumference should have an extra-long measuring tape.

Etiology

Although the basis of obesity (positive energy balance) could not be simpler, the factors affecting this energy imbalance are varied and complex. These factors include genetic, metabolic, and hormonal influences (19) that likely predispose some persons to obesity and may set the range of possible weights that an individual can achieve. Although it is likely that behavioral factors, such as increased portion sizes and decreased activity (20–22), are responsible for the increased prevalence of obesity, up to 50% to 70% of the variance in body weight in any one individual is accounted for by genetic factors (23,24). More than 300 genes have been linked to obesity, but single-gene mutations (eg, leptin deficiency) are extremely rare in human obesity (25). A genetic predisposition does not preclude clinically meaningful weight loss but does suggest that equivalent changes in eating and activity will produce different results among those of varying genotypes.

Treatment

Treatment of obesity is largely based on BMI and comorbidities (Figure 1.1) (26). Although behavioral approaches are used across the BMI continuum, pharmacological and surgical treatments are indicated among those with higher BMIs who have previously attempted more conservative approaches. It is worth repeating that small weight losses result in big improvements in the health profile, and that losing 5% to 10% of one's total body weight can result in clinically significant changes (3). It is this fact that makes the clini-

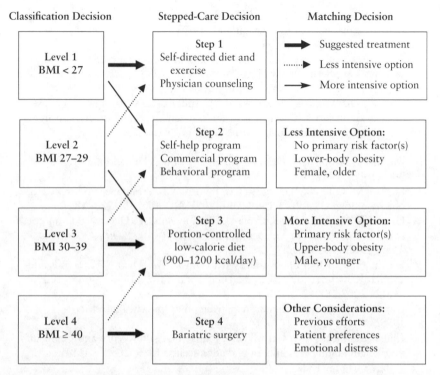

Figure 1.1. Model of Treatment for Obesity

Reprinted with permission from Wadden TA, Brownell KD, Foster GD. Obesity: responding to the global epidemic. *J Consult Clin Psychol.* 2002;70:510–525. Copyright © 2002 by the American Psychological Association.

cian's role so important. Independent of etiology, treatment is largely based on making environmental changes. It is in the clinician's purview, therefore, to help the obese patient to make lifestyle changes that may result in weight loss, and therefore, better health. The remainder of this book is devoted to the challenge of helping obese patients eat less and move more in an environment that encourages otherwise.

References

1. Fontaine KR, Redden DT, Wang C, Westfall AO, Allison DB. Years of life lost due to obesity. *JAMA.* 2003;289:187–193.
2. Calle EE, Rodriguez C, Walker-Thurmond K, Thun MJ. Overweight, obesity, and mortality from cancer in a prospectively studied cohort of U.S. adults. *N Engl J Med.* 2003;348:1625–1638.

3. National Institutes of Health. Clinical guidelines on the identification, evaluation, and treatment of overweight and obesity in adults—the evidence report. *Obes Res.* 1998;6:51S–209S.

4. Field AE, Barnoya J, Colditz GA. Epidemiology and health and economic consequences of obesity. In: Wadden TA, Stunkard AJ, eds. *Handbook of Obesity Treatment.* New York, NY: Guilford Press; 2002:3–18.

5. Wadden TA, Womble LG, Stunkard AJ, Anderson DA. Psychosocial consequences of obesity and weight loss. In: Wadden TA, Stunkard AJ, editors. *Handbook of Obesity Treatment.* New York, NY: Guilford Press; 2002:144–169.

6. Kushner R, Foster GD. Obesity and quality of life. *Nutrition.* 2000;16:947–952.

7. Flegal KM, Carroll MD, Ogden CL, Johnson CL. Prevalence and trends in obesity among US adults, 1999–2000. *JAMA.* 2002;288:1723–1727.

8. Flegal KM, Carroll MD, Kuczmarski RJ, Johnson CL. Overweight and obesity in the United States: prevalence and trends, 1960–1994. *Int J Obes Relat Metab Disord.* 1998;22:39–47.

9. Freedman DS, Khan LK, Serdula MK, Galuska DA, Dietz WH. Trends and correlates of class 3 obesity in the United States from 1990 through 2000. *JAMA.* 2002;288:1758–1761.

10. Foreyt J, Goodrick K. The ultimate triumph of obesity. *Lancet.* 1995;346:134–135.

11. Ogden CL, Flegal KM, Carroll MD, Johnson CL. Prevalence and trends in overweight among US children and adolescents, 1999–2000. *JAMA.* 2002;288:1728–1732.

12. World Health Organization. *Obesity: Preventing and Managing the Global Epidemic: Report of a WHO Consultation on Obesity.* Geneva, Switzerland: World Health Organization; 1998.

13. US Department of Health and Human Services, Public Health Service, Office of the Surgeon General. *Surgeon General's Call to Action to Prevent and Decrease Overweight and Obesity.* Rockville, Md: US Department of Health and Human Services; 2001.

14. Metropolitan Life Insurance Company. Metropolitan height and weight standards. *Statistical Bulletin of New York Metlife Insurance Company.* 1983;64:2–9.

15. Harrison GG. Height-weight tables. *Ann Intern Med.* 1985;103:989–994.

16. National Institutes of Health, National Heart, Lung, and Blood Institute. NHLBI Education Initiative. *The Practical Guide: Identification, Evaluation, and Treatment of Overweight and Obesity in Adults.* 2000. NIH Publication No. 00-4084. Available at: http://www.nhlbi.nih.gov/guidelines/obesity/prctgd_c.pdf. Accessed June 18, 2003.

17. Kissebah AH, Vydelingum N, Murray R, Evans DJ, Hartz AJ, Kalkhoff RK, Adams PW. Relation of body fat distribution to metabolic complications of obesity. *J Clin Endocrinol Metab.* 1982;54:254–260.

18. Lapidus L, Bengtsson B, Larsson B, Pennert K, Rybo E, Sjostrom D. Distribution of adipose tissue and risk of cardiovascular disease and death: a 12-year

follow-up of participants in the population study of women in Gothenburg, Sweden. *BMJ*. 1984;289:1261–1263.

19. Korner J, Aronne LJ. The emerging science of body weight regulation and its impact on obesity treatment. *J Clin Invest*. 2003;111:565–570.

20. Nielson SJ, Popkin BM. Patterns and trends in food portion sizes, 1977–1998. *JAMA*. 2003;289:450–453.

21. Foster GD, Phelan S. Environmental challenges and assessment. In: Berndanier C, ed. *Handbook of Nutrition and Food*. Boca Raton, Fla: CRC Press; 2001:773–785.

22. Rolls BJ. The supersizing of America: portion size and the obesity epidemic. *Nutr Today*. 2003;38:42–53.

23. Segal NL, Allison DB. Twins and virtual twins: bases of relative body weight revisited. *Int J Obes Relat Metab Disord*. 2002;26:437–441.

24. Comuzzie AJ. The genetic contribution to human obesity: the dissection of a complex phenotype. In: Johnston FE, Foster GD, eds. *Obesity, Growth and Development*. London, England: Smith-Gordon & Co; 2001:21–36.

25. Chagnon YC, Rankinen T, Snyder EE, Weisnagel SJ, Pérusse L, Bouchard C. The human obesity gene map: the 2002 update. *Obes Res*. 2003;11:313–367.

26. Wadden TA, Brownell KD, Foster GD. Obesity: responding to the global epidemic. *J Consult Clin Psychol*. 2002;70:510–525.

Chapter 2

Assessment

PART A. Overview

Sachiko T. St. Jeor, PhD, RD,
Holly Herzog, MS, RD, and Doina Kulick, MD

As the rates of obesity and concomitant risk have increased, obesity as a disease has received more recognition. This has helped to underscore the importance of good nutrition assessment and screening for improved health outcomes. During a patient's hospital stay, the effect of weight should be considered when medications are prescribed, when diseases are being treated, and when referral options are being discussed. In the outpatient setting, where the distinction of obesity as a metabolic disorder (1), particularly metabolic syndrome (2), plays a large part in treatment plans, obesity has also created new opportunities for reimbursement. The ICD-9-CM Codes for Obesity (278.00 Obesity, Unspecified, or 278.01 Extreme or Morbid Obesity), as determined by the treating physician, are frequently not covered, or reimbursed by insurance companies. The new code for the metabolic syndrome (277.7) is more successful in terms of reimbursement; also, the codes for associated manifestations, such as cardiovascular disease (CVD) (414.00–414.05), diabetes (250.01–250.03), and dyslipidemia (272.0–272.4) are more successfully covered and subsequently reimbursed (3).

Medical record documentation is essential for maintaining communication among health care professionals about patient care and can take different forms. A variety of formats are available to document in the medical chart; the most common style of progress note continues to be the Subjective, Objective, Assessment, and Plan (SOAP) note (4). The purpose of this chapter is to review assessment of obesity using the SOAP note as a guide. Most SOAP notes do not address obesity as a central theme. Therefore, clinicians do not often associate the presence of obesity with concomitant complaints; they also do not often consider weight loss as the treatment to reduce associated risks. The following discussion addresses aspects of a SOAP note that include obesity as a major disease entity. The Practical Applications sections of this chapter will explore the SOAP method in more depth in different settings.

SOAP Note

Subjective

Chief Complaint.   Depending on what the patient reports as the primary reason for the initial visit (eg, dyspnea upon exertion, uncontrolled diabetes, or weight loss for an event), the chief complaint may or may not be related to weight loss.

Medical History and Current Health Status.   Any reference to diseases (eg, sleep apnea, gallbladder disease, eating disorders, or psychosocial history) should be addressed in this section. Allergies, use of medications and supplements, bowel irregularities, or other reported factors that might affect body weight should be included.

Weight History.   Information on weight history should include the following:

- Current weight
- Weight 6, 12, and 60 months ago
- Highest adult body weight and when the patient had it
- Lowest adult body weight and when the patient had it
- Goal weight
- Critical periods for weight gain
- Perceived reasons for weight gain or loss

Weight Loss History.   The patient's dieting history, a self-evaluation of the patient's risk for further weight gain, and the patient's ability to maintain weight should be included (5,6).

Dietary Intake.   The patient is prompted to recall a typical daily intake.

Family History. Both diseases and weights of family members should be included.

Social History. Support networks and cultural factors should be identified. This provides important information for the assessment of perceived behavioral and psychological barriers to, and facilitators of, change.

Lifestyle and Behavioral Factors. Usual physical activity, determination of goals both long-term (1 year) and short-term (3 to 6 months), readiness for weight-loss interventions, and any insight into how to achieve and maintain long-term compliance should be identified.

Objective

This section includes factual information that can be documented and that is pertinent to the current assessment, such as the following:

- An accurate weight (taken in light clothing, without shoes, with a beam-balance, calibrated scale)
- A correct height measurement (taken by a stadiometer or wall-mounted height board)
- Body mass index (BMI) (calculated by weight in kg/ht in m^2). Note the National Institutes of Health (NIH) guidelines for underweight (BMI < 18.5), normal weight (BMI = 18.5 to 24.9), overweight (BMI = 25.0 to 29.9), obesity class I (BMI = 30.0 to 34.9), obesity class II (BMI = 35.0 to 39.9), and extreme obesity or class III (BMI ≥ 40) (7,8).
- Waist circumference. Although controversy exists about how to correctly measure the waist, the point at the iliac crest has been recommended by NIH and appears to give the most reproducible results (7,8).
- Any pertinent laboratory tests or measurements
- Medications, both prescription and over-the-counter (vitamin and herbal)

Review psychological or behavioral tests, such as the Diet Readiness (9,10), General Well-Being Schedule (9,11,12) and Readiness to Change data (13). Measures of body composition can be helpful but are expensive. Dual Energy X-ray Absorptiometry (DXA), computed tomography (CT scans), magnetic resonance imaging (MRI), and skinfolds can also be used, if appropriate and available (14,15). Bioimpedance may provide some balance between reliability and cost (16).

Assessment

Based on the subjective and objective findings, the assessment portion of the SOAP note confirms the medical diagnosis provided by the treating physician. The patient's adherence potential to treatment should be considered and then appropriate medical nutrition therapy interventions are recommended. The assessment should include the following items:

- All comorbidities, such as metabolic syndrome, type 2 diabetes, cardiovascular disease, osteoarthritis, gallbladder disease, sleep apnea, and respiratory problems, as well as a history of cancers of the breast, colon, prostate, and endometrium. Not only do these risk factors affect treatment and/or expected outcomes, but, unlike obesity, these risk factors are usually reimbursable.
- Whether weight is exacerbating the health problems and therefore should be treated more aggressively.
- Whether the use of a specific kind of diet is warranted.
- Whether any medication is potentially causing weight gain.
- Any concern that weight loss will have adverse effects on binge eating, depression, anxiety, or stress; quality of life issues.
- The reasons for physical inactivity.
- Exclusion criteria for weight reduction that would indicate postponement of weight-loss treatment and recommendations for weight maintenance or prevention of further weight gain. Such criteria would include pregnancy, lactation, unstable mental illness, unstable medical conditions, and chronic debilitating diseases.
- Criteria that require further consideration by the physician, such as cholelithiasis or age 80 years or older.
- Energy expenditure and suggested energy deficit (see "Assessing Energy Balance" section of this chapter).

Plan

After careful assessment, the individual is given a personalized plan developed using the current practice of weight management. This plan should include the following:

- Referrals (eg, to psychologists, exercise physiologists, group education)
- Nutrition intervention
- Physical activity regimen
- Suggested behavioral modification
- Short-term goals
- Monitoring and evaluation

Assessing Energy Balance

Total energy expenditure (TEE) should be estimated to counsel patients on the level of energy intake that is needed for weight maintenance and/or prevention of weight gain or regain. Although indirect calorimetry is the most desirable to calculate the resting energy expenditure (REE), it is not always available. Therefore, many predictive formulas and methods (17) have been used to estimate basal energy expenditure (BEE) or REE. Clinicians have debated the accuracy and practical application of predictive formulas, particularly as it relates to obesity. The most commonly used equations are the Harris Benedict Formula (for BEE) and the Mifflin-St. Jeor Formula (for REE, or 10% above BEE). Recently, the Macronutrient Panel of the Institute of Medicine (18) has made the following recommendations for estimating TEE:

- Men ≥ 19 years:

  TEE = 864 − 9.72 × age (y) + PA × [14.2 × wt (kg) + 503 × ht (m)]

- Women ≥ 19 years:

  TEE = 387 − 7.31 × age (y) + PA × [10.9 × wt (kg) + 660.7 × ht (m)]

  Where: PA = physical activity coefficient.

These recommendations make adjustments for level of PA as follows: sedentary (≥1.0 to <1.4); low active (≥1.4 to <1.6); active (≥1.6 to <1.9); and very active (≥1.9 to <2.5), to be used in the equations (19). Adjustments are also made for kcal/day, recommended for age and sex: ±7 for women and ±10 for men, for each year above or below age 30 years.

Recently a new hand-held device for measuring metabolic rate and oxygen consumption (MedGem) was approved as a medical device by the Food and Drug Administration. This more convenient technology allows clinicians to measure in a reliable manner rather than estimate REE (20).

Creating an Energy Deficit

Once the TEE is calculated, current guidelines recommend an energy deficit of −250 to −1,000 kcal/day in dietary intake, to induce weight loss of approximately −0.5 to −2.0 lb per week (7,8).

Another dilemma is the accuracy in calculating energy intake. Clinical assessment of energy intake and eating behaviors is a practiced skill. Assessment of food intake is difficult at best, given that calories in actual meals can be difficult to calculate accurately, portion sizes must be estimated, snacking episodes must be counted, and environmental influences must be considered. Quick screens (21) and computerized programs (22) are available to assist with the analysis, but cost, time, and ease of application may be obstacles. Ultimately, the clinical professional uses a predictive equation to estimate TEE, a best-guess effort to calculate energy intake, and years of professional experience to adjust either calculation as the patient is assessed in follow-up.

Conclusion

Good screening and assessment skills are the keys to successful obesity treatment. Professionals should recommend diet and physical activity to reverse the epidemic of obesity. Although weight management for already overweight and obese adults is critically important, early intervention and preventive efforts (including weight maintenance strategies) for children and adults at risk are equally as important in helping to improve the health of individuals. Clinicians have the opportunity to lead the way in improving assessments so that interventions will be more effective and cost efficient in the long run.

References

1. Blackburn GL, Ishikawa M, Miller D. Biomarkers to characterize various types of obesity. In: St. Jeor ST, ed. *Obesity Assessment: Tools, Methods, Interpretations*. New York: Chapman & Hall; 1997:101–113.
2. Executive Summary of the Third Report of the National Cholesterol Education Program (NCEP) Expert Panel on Detection, Evaluation, and Treatment of High Blood Cholesterol in Adults (Adult Treatment Panel III). *JAMA*. 2001;285:2486–2497.
3. Hart AC, Hopkins CA, eds. *2003 ICD-9-CM Professional for Physicians: International Classification of Diseases, 9th revision, Clinical Modification*: Effective October 1, 2002-September 30, 2003. 6th ed. Salt Lake City, Utah: Ingenix; 2002.
4. Guild M. Clinical Nutrition: An Interactive Approach. Items To Include in SOAP Notes. College of Allied Health, University of Oklahoma; 1998. Available at: http://w3.uokhsc.edu/mguild/cn2case/instructions.html. Accessed October 8, 2002.
5. St. Jeor ST, Brunner RL, Harrington ME, Scott BJ, Daugherty SA, Cutter GR, Brownell KD, Dyer AR, Foreyt JP. A classification system to evaluate weight maintainers, gainers and losers. *J Am Diet Assoc*. 1997;97:481–488.
6. St. Jeor ST, Brunner RL, Harrington ME, Scott BJ, Cutter GR, Brownell KD, Dyer AR, Foreyt JP. Who are the weight maintainers? *Obes Res*. 1995;3(suppl 2):249S–259S.
7. National Heart, Lung, and Blood Institute and National Institute of Diabetes and Digestive and Kidney Diseases, National Institutes of Health. *Clinical Guidelines on the Identification, Evaluation, and Treatment of Overweight*

and Obesity in Adults. Bethesda, Md: National Institutes of Health; 1998:228. NIH Publication No. 98-4083.

8. National Heart, Lung, and Blood Institute, National Institutes of Health, and North American Association for the Study of Obesity. *The Practical Guide: Identification, Evaluation, and Treatment of Overweight and Obesity in Adults.* Bethesda, Md: National Institutes of Health; 2000:77. NIH Publication No. 00-4084.

9. *Weighing the Options: Criteria for Evaluating Weight Management Programs.* Washington, DC: National Academy Press; 1995:282.

10. Brownell KD. Dieting readiness. *Weight Control Digest.* 1990;1:5–10.

11. Miller GD, Harrington ME. General well-being schedule. In: St. Jeor ST, ed. *Obesity Assessment: Tools, Methods, Interpretations.* New York, NY: Chapman and Hall; 1997:465–470,857–863.

12. The general well-being schedule. In: McDowell I, Newell C. *Measuring Health: A Guide to Rating Scales and Questionnaires.* New York, NY: Oxford University Press; 1987:125–133.

13. Prochaska J, DiClimente CC. Transtheoretical approach: toward a more integrative model of change. *Psychotherapy.* 1982;20:161.

14. Van Loan MD. The how and why of body composition assessment. In: Berdanier CD, Feldman EB, Flatt WP, St. Jeor ST, ed. *Handbook of Nutrition and Food.* Boca Raton, Fla: CRC Press; 2002:637–656.

15. Scott BJ. Frame size, circumferences and skinfolds. In: Berdanier CD, Feldman EB, Flatt WP, St. Jeor ST, eds. *Handbook of Nutrition and Food.* Boca Raton, Fla: CRC Press; 2002:657–672.

16. St. Jeor ST, ed. *Obesity Assessment: Tools, Methods, Interpretations.* New York, NY: Chapman and Hall; 1997.

17. Mifflin MD, St. Jeor ST, Hill LA, Scott BJ, Daugherty SA, Koh YO. A new predictive equation for resting energy expenditure in healthy individuals. *Am J Clin Nutr.* 1990;51:241–247.

18. Institute of Medicine, National Academy of Sciences. *Dietary Reference Intakes. Energy, Carbohydrate, Fiber, Fat, Fatty Acids, Cholesterol, Protein and Amino Acids.* Prepublication copy. Washington DC: National Academy of Sciences; September 2002.

19. Almeida MJ, Blair SN. Energy assessment: physical activity. In: Berdanier CD, Feldman EB, Flatt WP, St. Jeor ST, eds. *Handbook of Nutrition and Food.* Boca Raton, Fla: CRC Press; 2002:737–755.

20. Nieman DC, Trone GA, Austin MD. A new hand-held device for measuring resting energy expenditure and oxygen consumption. *J Am Diet Assoc.* 2003;103:588–593.

21. Gans K, Ross E, Barner C, Wylie-Rosett J, McMurray J, Eaton C. REAP and WAVE: new tools to rapidly assess/discuss nutrition with patients. *J Nutr.* 2003;133:556S–562S.

22. Ashley JM, Grossbauer S. Computerized nutrient analysis systems. In: Berdanier CD, Feldman EB, Flatt WP, St. Jeor ST, eds. *Handbook of Nutrition and Food.* Boca Raton, Fla: CRC Press: 2002;559–565.

PART B. Practical Applications: Inpatient

Siri Sirichanvimol, MS, RD

Given the increasing prevalence and associated morbidity of obesity, it is no surprise that clinicians are encountering more obese individuals in the hospital setting. Approximately 25% to 35% of hospitalized patients are overweight or obese (1–3). This poses clinical challenges for practitioners, because routine hospital care can become complicated, especially for severely obese individuals. Increased incidences of insulin resistance and glucose intolerance, infection, bacteremia, sepsis, prolonged mechanical ventilation, and mortality have been identified among hospitalized patients who are obese. Additionally, obese postoperative patients may be more likely than nonobese patients to develop wound dehiscence, nosocomial infections, respiratory complications, and delayed cardiac recuperation (4–7). The purpose of this Practical Applications section is to review principles and practices of assessing obese patients in a hospital setting.

Metabolic Changes Associated With Obesity

There is a cycle of conditions and treatment that exacerbates both the obesity and the associated risks. For example, obese patients are often insulin resistant at baseline. This condition can lead to glucose intolerance and hyperinsulinemia, hyperlipidemia, coronary artery disease, and hypertension. The presence of severe illness or infection can exacerbate insulin resistance, which leads to an intolerance of large volumes of intravenous dextrose solutions and hyperglycemia and is unresponsive to routine treatment. Elevated serum glucose levels increase the susceptibility to infection, impair the immune function, and delay wound healing. Hyperinsulinemia may occur or may be exacerbated, which leads to salt and water retention, causing fluid overload. Such a condition places the patient at risk for pulmonary edema and congestive heart failure. Excess glucose infusion can increase carbon dioxide production, thus impairing respiratory function or delaying ventilatory weaning in an obese patient with underlying respiratory compromise. Hepatic dysfunction, which is commonly associated with critical illness, is of concern because of the already increased incidence of fatty liver in this population. Finally, excess caloric infusion can promote hepatic dysfunction and lipid infusion intolerance, as reflected by elevated liver function tests, hypercholesterolemia, and hypertriglyceridemia (8–10).

Critically Ill Obese Patients

Critical illness, regardless of body weight, increases protein requirements. These increased protein requirements are caused by the use of lean body mass as an endogenous energy source that results from hypercatabolism, increased energy expenditure, and protein turnover. Malnutrition can develop rapidly if protein requirements are not met by exogenous sources (8,10). A study by Jeevanandam et al suggests that more protein and less fat per kilogram of body weight are mobilized in obese, critically ill trauma patients, whereas increased fat oxidation and decreased carbohydrate and protein oxidation occur in nonobese patients (11). Although more studies on this topic are needed, the fact remains that exogenous fuel (particularly protein) is required to combat protein catabolism and to maintain lean body mass and visceral protein stores—no matter what the body mass index (BMI) (10,12).

Delayed nutrition support sometimes occurs because of the perception that obese patients can mobilize endogenous lipid as an abundant and sufficient fuel source. However, the ability of the critically ill obese patient to sufficiently mobilize stored fat is still a matter of debate (9).

Energy and Protein Requirements for Critically Ill Obese Patients

Protein administration of 1.5 to 2.0 g/kg ideal body weight (IBW) per day or 1.25 g/kg actual body weight (ABW) per day, in patients without renal or hepatic dysfunction, appears to maintain positive nitrogen balance in obese patients on hypocaloric regimens (8–10,13–16). However, it may not be possible to achieve positive nitrogen balance during the first 2 weeks of critical illness in any patient after severe trauma, especially if an anabolic steroid is administered. At such times, the goal is to minimize nitrogen losses. It is unclear whether providing more protein during this time improves nitrogen balance in the metabolically stressed patient. Studies on optimal protein intake in the critically ill obese patient are lacking (10).

Maximizing protein sparing is also crucial to effective nutrition support. The infusion of amino acids without dextrose or lipid will not prevent nitrogen loss. The addition of carbohydrate and fat in total parenteral nutrition (TPN) has actually been shown to improve protein sparing. It is theorized that once glycogen stores have been rapidly depleted in a stressed patient, the body will rely on gluconeogenesis to provide fuel to support the immune system, wound healing, and the peripheral nervous system (9).

The amount of nonprotein calories necessary to maximize protein sparing is unknown. An early study by Elwyn et al reported that nitrogen preservation was achieved with higher energy administration, but the effect was blunted once energy delivery exceeded 60% of resting energy expenditure (REE) (17). It is not generally advisable to exceed this amount in non-burn patients, considering the potentially hazardous effects of overfeeding. Published recommendations for nonprotein calories vary widely, from a maximum of 25 kcal/kg ABW (or 36 kcal/kg IBW) to 14 kcal/kg ABW (or 22 kcal/kg IBW) (8–10,12). The use of 21 or 22 total kcal (protein and nonprotein)/kg ABW has been suggested as a quick estimate of energy expenditure in ventilator-dependent obese patients (11). Dickerson et al recently published a study reporting that patients receiving <20 total kcal (protein and nonprotein)/kg ABW had a shorter ICU stay, fewer days of antibiotic treatment, and fewer days of mechanical ventilation than obese patients receiving ≥20 total kcal/kg ABW. The goal protein intake for both groups in this study was 2 g of protein/kg IBW/d (10).

Estimating Energy Expenditure in Critical Care

There is a general lack of agreement on nutrition intervention in the hospitalized obese population. The goal of nutrition in this setting is essentially to support the preservation of lean body mass (LBM) by maintaining or promoting positive nitrogen balance, promoting wound healing and recovery, and preventing complications associated with overfeeding (10,11, 18). The best method by which this is accomplished is still being debated. Many facilities do not have access to a metabolic cart (9,12), for indirect calorimetry (the gold standard to estimate energy expenditure). In the absence of such a device, clinicians rely on predictive formulas (19). However, critical illness adds another complication to the questions of accuracy for energy expenditure equations. A stress factor ranging from 1.0 to 1.5 has been applied to the Harris Benedict formula to predict total energy expenditure (TEE) (9,11,18,20). The literature reports conflicting results. For instance, Leibel et al found that the use of actual body weight in the Harris Benedict formula tended to overestimate energy expenditure in nonobese as well as obese patients (21). Ireton-Jones et al advocate the use of ABW over ideal body weight (IBW) and developed a regression equation for obese energy expenditure (OEE) and ventilator-dependent expenditure (VEE) (22,23). Trombley et al reported the highest level of correlation between calculated energy expenditure and measured expenditure, using IBW and adjusted body weight in the Harris Benedict equation, with no stress factor (12). Glynn et al compared adjusted body weight (adjusting for changes in fluid) and an average weight (AVG = 50% between ABW and IBW) and found that the Harris Benedict equation, using average weight with a stress factor of 1.3, accurately predicted measured energy expenditure in the critically ill obese (18).

With so many variations in the method of calculating energy expenditure, practitioners will have to rely on clinical judgment with institutional guidelines when recommending protein and energy needs for obese patients. To make matters more difficult, obtaining accurate weights for a critically ill obese patient can be difficult because of fluid issues (eg, edema, ascites, anasarca, fluid resuscitation, and diuresis). Obtaining admission weight and tracking daily weights in critical patients may help clinicians to determine a more accurate weight (24). In the absence of a metabolic cart for indirect calorimetry, quick estimates of 20 to 22 total kcal/kg ABW and 1.5 g of protein/kg IBW may be a practical starting point. Predictive formulas can be used to double-check estimated ranges and could be useful when taking into consideration various stress factors.

Case Studies

Two case studies of hospitalized obese patients are presented here. The first focuses on maintaining lean tissue and whether obesity treatment is appropriate. The second addresses weight loss directly.

Case Study. Critically Ill Hospitalized Patient

Sam Jones is a 59-year-old man, 69 inches, 210 lb, IBW 160 lb, and BMI = 31. He was admitted for chronic obstructive pulmonary disease (COPD) exacerbation, fever, and gastrointestinal bleeding. When admitted to the intensive care unit, he was in respiratory distress and required intubation. Fever and acute gastrointestinal bleeding were worked up. Medical history included sleep apnea, congestive heart failure (for which he was prescribed a chronic diuretic and steroid therapy), a myocardial infarction 2 years past, type 2 diabetes controlled with a combination of insulin and sulfonylureas, and hypertension controlled with an ace inhibitor. The patient had several admissions to the hospital for COPD exacerbation and respiratory infections requiring antibiotic treatment. He was NPO since his admission 2 days earlier. Total parenteral nutrition (TPN) was ordered.

Most clinicians will try to adhere to the standard 30% lipid, 20% protein, and 50% carbohydrate ratios for TPN. However, in the case of an obese patient with diabetes and poor insulin sensitivity who is moderately stressed and on steroid therapy, 40% carbohydrate and 30% to 40% lipid or 20% to 30% protein is appropriate. If liver function tests and triglycerides continue to increase, then the lipid will have to be reduced. Therefore, baseline assessment and frequent follow-up lab tests are essential to designing TPN that is optimal for the patient.

Overfeeding is a major concern for any critically ill patient but especially so for an obese patient. However, weight loss during this critical time may not be appropriate. Providing 20 to 25 kcal/kg ABW may be sufficient to meet required needs and to maintain weight. Because fluid weight often changes during diuresis, it may be prudent to readjust calories as fluid is lost. It is helpful to monitor the daily weights and the total intake and output (specifically urine output) and to document them in the chart.

SOAP Note

Subjective

Patient is intubated, unable to interview; therefore, information typically listed under "Subjective" can be found under "Objective."

Objective

A 59-year-old man admitted with COPD exacerbation, respiratory distress requiring intubation, fever, and gastrointestinal bleeding.

Past medical history: COPD, congestive heart failure, sleep apnea, type 2 diabetes controlled with insulin and oral hypoglycemic agent, hypertension, and myocardial infarction (2 years ago).

Anthropometrics: 69 inches, IBW: 160 lb ±10%, current weight: 210 lb (131% IBW), BMI = 31, unknown weight history.

Labs: BUN: 26; glucose: 256; AST: 44; ALT: 49; total cholesterol: 265; LDL-C: 195; HDL-C: 38; triglycerides: 178; albumin: 2.9; hgb/hct: 12.2/36.6; CR: 0.9.

Medications: Chronic antihypertensive, diuretic, and steroid treatment. Periodic antibiotic use.

Assessment

Patient exhibits moderate obesity, based on his BMI of 31. Patient is currently at moderate to high nutritional risk, secondary to albumin of 2.9 (may be falsely low due to edema and fluid overload), weight status (131% IBW), respiratory distress, medical history, and NPO status. Patient requires TPN. Elevated liver function tests and triglyceride levels may be related to chronic steroid, diuretic, antihypertensive, and frequent antibiotic treatment. Elevated levels may also be reflective of dietary noncompliance and obesity. Slightly high BUN may be due to diuretic treatment, because serum creatinine is within normal limits and urine output is good. Low albumin may be secondary to fluid status and stress and is not a good test of protein status. Therefore, a pre-albumin level that can be tracked often may be more indicative of visceral protein status. The patient's low hgb/hct is mostly likely due to gastrointestinal bleeding.

Estimated needs for TPN: Recommend the following for metabolic stress and preservation of lean body mass:
1,900 to 2,090 kcal (20 to 22kcal/kg ABW)
108 to 144 g protein (1.5 to 2.0 g Pro/kg IBW)
2,375 cc fluid (25 cc/kg fluid restriction per physician)

Plan

1. Patient is NPO. Recommend TPN using calculations above.
2. Recommend daily weights during diuresis.
3. Suggest prealbumin level every Tuesday and Friday until discharge.
4. Glucose monitoring every 4 hours with insulin coverage, with adjustment of insulin in TPN as appropriate.
5. Monitor input and output, weight changes, and electrolytes, and adjust TPN accordingly.
6. Please order liver function and triglyceride tests with other labs before TPN initiation and daily after TPN infusion reaches goal.

Education: Nutrition education in Mr. Jones's case is for the caretakers, not Mr. Jones. Education will be minimal, at best, because of the limited amount of time that the caretaker is available on the patient care unit and the volume of patients who require intervention by the dietitian. Education in a hospital setting should address the current medical/surgical issue. However, on discharge, written education can be provided to address long-term dietary issues. Referral to an outpatient dietitian can be of great benefit. Communication between the dietitian and the home care attendant may improve the long-term management of both diabetes and obesity. In-depth counseling is not practical or possible in a hospital setting in most circumstances.

Case Study. Noncritical Hospitalized Patient

Susan Jones, a 55-year-old woman, 67 inches, 210 lb, was admitted for knee replacement. Medical history includes coronary artery disease (CAD) and high cholesterol, but she denies any liver or renal disease. She will be discharged to home when she is stabilized and can tolerate a regular diet postoperatively.

SOAP Note

Subjective

Patient was admitted for knee replacement. Medical history includes CAD and high cholesterol.

Weight history: Patient is currently at highest adult weight. Her lowest body weight was 145 lb before her first child was born. Patient has gained 20 lb with each of her two pregnancies and 30 pounds postmenopause. She states that she would like to lose weight now. She has tried many different diets, including a liquid formula, Weight Watchers, and amphetamines.

Dietary intake: Patient cooks for family and tends to nibble in kitchen between meals. She partakes in no physical activity. Restaurant eating includes "too much bread."

Family history: Father has hypertension and CAD; maternal grandmother has diabetes. Mother is obese but currently has no diabetes.

Medications: None. Occasionally takes a multivitamin and calcium.

Objective

A 55-year-old woman who is just postsurgery for knee replacement.

Anthropometrics: Patient is 67 inches. IBW: 140 lb ± 10%. Current weight of 210 lb is 150% IBW. BMI = 33.

Labs: Cholesterol: 219; HDL-C: 42; triglyceride: 195; glucose: 111; blood pressure: 138/88. Waist circumference could not be measured because of the patient's inability to stand.

Assessment

Patient is an obese, pleasant woman with metabolic syndrome and a desire to lose weight. Family history of diabetes and cardiovascular disease and her obesity put her at risk for development of diabetes and heart disease. She understands the basics of a healthy weight-loss diet but has difficulty adhering to any one diet. She had very little physical activity before surgery secondary to knee pain. She seems receptive to weight loss now, likely because of concern for her health. Her estimated caloric need for weight loss: 20 kcal/kg IBW = 1,300 kcal, but suggest an increase to 1,500.

Plan

1. Recommendation: continue low-cholesterol, low-fat diet during hospitalization.
2. Discharge diet: 1,500 kcal/day, low-fat diet, with a significant increase of vegetables.
3. Encourage compliance with dietary principles and behavioral changes.
4. Refer to outpatient education for follow-up (or http://www. eatright.org).

Education: Verbal and written counseling provided regarding 1,500 kcal/day food pattern (50% of meals as vegetables) and portion control. Discussed limiting access to snack foods. Patient will consider over-the-counter formula as a meal replacement for lunch. Patient is able to plan meals using dietary pattern, but compliance with this regimen has not been good in the past. Patient would benefit from regular follow-up sessions with outpatient dietitian for support and further education.

Final Note

Clinical nutrition assessment of the obese hospitalized patient has a different focus from that of a nonhospitalized individual. Although level of obesity may exacerbate the presenting diagnosis, it is seldom the primary concern. However, nutrition intervention is crucial to support recovery for all patients, regardless of their adiposity. Furthermore, clinicians generally agree that weight stability or some weight loss during hospitalization is helpful in improving health outcomes and therefore should be addressed in all assessments. Controversy exists over predicting estimated needs and the recommendations for caloric and protein requirements in obese patients.

References

1. Herbert HB, Feinleib M, McNamara PM, Castelli WP. Obesity as an independent risk factor for cardiovascular disease: a 26-year follow-up of participants in the Framingham Heart Study. *Circulation*. 1983;67:968–977.
2. Kamel HK, Iqbal MA. Body mass index and mortality among hospitalized patients. *Arch Intern Med*. 2001;161:1459–1460.
3. Potter JF, Schafer DF, Bohi RL. In-hospital mortality as a function of body mass index: an age-dependent variable. *J Gerontol*. 1988;43:M59–M63.
4. Choban PS, Heckler R, Burge J, Flancbaum L. Increased incidence of nosocomial infections in obese surgical patients. *Am Surg*. 1995;61:1001–1005.
5. Choban PS, Weireter LJ, Maynes C. Obesity and increased mortality in blunt trauma. *J Trauma*. 1991;31:1253–1257.
6. Drenick EJ, Bale GS, Seltzer F, Johnson DG. Excessive mortality and causes of death in morbidly obese men. *JAMA*. 1980;243:443–445.
7. Mathison CJ. Skin and wound care challenges in the hospitalized morbidly obese patient. *J Wound Ostomy Continence Nurs*. 2003;30:78–83.
8. Choban PS, Flancbaum L. Nourishing the obese patient. *Clin Nutr*. 2000;19:305–311.
9. Shikora SA. Nutrition support for the obese patient. *Nutr Clin Care*. 1999; 2:230–238.
10. Dickerson RN, Boschert KJ, Kudsk KA, Brown RO. Hypocaloric enteral tube feeding in critically ill obese patients. *Nutrition*. 2002;18:241–246.
11. Jeevanandam M, Yound DH, Schiller WR. Obesity and the metabolic response to severe multiple trauma in man. *J Clin Invest*. 1991;87:262–269.
12. Trombley LE, Reinhard T, Klurfeld D. Energy expenditure in the critically ill obese patient. *Support Line*. 2001;32:18–24.
13. Choban PS, Burge JC, Scales D, Flancbaum L. Hypoenergetic nutrition support in hospitalized obese patients: a simplified method for clinical applications. *Am J Clin Nutr*.1997;66:546–550.
14. Baxter JK, Bistrian BR. Moderate hypocaloric parenteral nutrition in the critically ill, obese patient. *Nutr Clin Pract*. 1989;4:133–135.
15. Dickerson RN, Rosato EF, Mullen JL. Net protein anabolism with hypocaloric parenteral nutrition in obese stressed patients. *Am J Clin Nutr*. 1986;44: 747–755.
16. Burge JC, Goon A, Choban PS, Flancbaum L. Efficacy of hypocaloric total parenteral nutrition in hospitalized obese patients: a prospective, double-blind randomized trial. *J Parenter Enteral Nutr*. 1994;18:203–207.
17. Elwyn DH, Kinney JM, Askanazi J. Energy expenditure in surgical patients. *Surg Clin North Am*. 1981;61:545–556.
18. Glynn CC, Greene GW, Winkler MF, Albina JE. Predictive vs. measured energy expenditure using limits-of-agreement analysis in hospitalized, obese patients. *J Parenter Enteral Nutr*. 1999;23:147–154.
19. Mifflin MD, St. Jeor ST, Hill LA, Scott BJ, Daugherty SA, Koh YO. A new predictive equation for resting energy expenditure in healthy individuals. *Am J Clin Nutr*. 1990;51:241–247.
20. Cutts ME, Dowdy RP, Ellersieck MR, Edes TE. Predicting energy needs in

ventilator-dependent critically ill patients: effect of adjusting weight for edema or adiposity. *Am J Clin Nutr.* 1997;66:1250–1256.

21. Leibel RL, Rosenbaum M, Hirsch J. Changes in resting energy expenditure resulting from altered weight. *N Engl J Med.* 1995;332:621–628.
22. Ireton-Jones CS, Turner WW Jr. Actual or ideal body weight: which should be used to predict energy expenditure? *J Am Diet Assoc.* 1991;91:193–195.
23. Ireton-Jones CS, Borman KR, Turner WW. Nutrition considerations in the management of ventilator-dependent patients. *Nutr Clin Pract.* 1993;8:60–64.
24. Hunter DC, Jaksic T, Lewis D, Benotti PN, Blackburn GL, Bistrian BR. Resting energy expenditure in the critically ill: estimations versus measurement. *Br J Surg.* 1988;75:875–878.

PART C. Practical Applications: Outpatient

Bonnie Taub-Dix, MA, RD, CDN

Unlike the practitioner completing an inpatient assessment, providers in the outpatient setting have the luxury of time—generally up to 1 hour. This allows the provider to conduct a more comprehensive assessment that includes environmental and cultural triggers, two pieces of the lifestyle puzzle that enhance patient-specific treatment (1). The luxury of time also affords the opportunity to design guidelines, rather than rules, that allow the client to become more involved in the process of lifestyle change. At times, therefore, a health care provider may be viewed as a teacher, a hand holder, a police officer, and even a warden. The provider-client team should examine decisions—such as what will work, how best to incorporate these changes, and whether such changes are realistic. The provider can set the stage and point the client in the right direction, but it is the client who ultimately must make the decision to change (2), and it is the client who must live with his or her choices. The purpose of this section is to describe the assessment tools—both formal and informal—that may assist the private practice practitioner in helping the client to reach his or her weight goals safely and effectively.

Before Consultation

A good nutrition assessment begins with the first telephone call. This is where the beginnings of a plan are formulated. Everything from educational needs to readiness to start, to level of illness, to payment information should be a part of the first telephone interaction. A critical component of any assessment is quite basic—listening. Listening is not a passive activity. From the first telephone call, when the health professional begins to assess the patient's level of literacy and his or her commitment, listening is a skill that is vital to clinical care (3). Having time to interpret and identify the meanings behind words and actions can help the clinician to establish a firmer relationship with the client. For example, is the client well versed in nutrition information yet lacking in the ability to apply such knowledge? The following section describes key areas to be assessed during the telephone contact.

Educational Needs

The first telephone call should yield information about the client's educational needs. Therefore, it is important for the provider to question the client if the information is not forthcoming. This previsit information gives the provider the opportunity to be ready with appropriate information, such as handouts on low-sodium foods or a list of calcium supplements, to be offered during the actual assessment.

If a client has attempted various diets in the past and understands the basics of dieting, perhaps the issue of emotional support should be explored. For example, if a client states, "My husband is very supportive; whenever I reach for a roll he pulls the breadbasket away from me," she may really be resentful and angry over her spouse's unsolicited control over her diet. In such a case, asking if such actions work to reduce her food intake can help to expose the more important issues. In turn, on that first visit, the provider and the client can discuss ways for the client to approach her husband on being more supportive. This change of direction, brought about by skilled listening, addresses a potentially big problem (support), helps to clarify an important part of food intake (who is ultimately responsible?) and creates solutions (such as asking her husband if it would be viable to take the bread basket away from the table) (4).

Readiness To Start

Another example of interpreting mixed messages concerns whether the client is actually ready to start a diet for weight loss. Is she consulting with you because a spouse or doctor has persuaded her to do so? Many individuals believe that they will receive nothing more from a dietitian than a sheet of paper with a rigid, unappealing dietary regimen to follow. It is helpful to dispel these myths immediately and to reduce unrealistic expectations. Reassure the client that no food is forbidden and that classifying food as "bad" or "good" is not useful. Remember, the more open a client is about eating habits (where, when, with whom, how much, and why), and the less threatened the client feels, the more the provider will be able to help (1–6).

Health Consequences

How weight loss and diet affect health outcomes depends on how sick a patient might be. Therefore, it is important to get an assessment of health status from a physician. Make it clear to the client that, as a nonphysician provider, you will work with the primary care physician (see Chapter 3: Clinical Monitoring). Make the patient a part of this process by requiring that information from the primary care physician—such as recent lab reports, physical notes, or results from any tests, (eg, bone density or stress tests)—be brought to the first visit. If the patient is unable to bring this medical information, obtain permission to contact the physician. Establishing relationships with physicians and other health professionals communicates to the patient that a cohesive team is working on his or her behalf (7,8).

Payment

It is critical to state how long the patient should plan to spend in your office and to be clear about the fee. Discuss insurance issues, whether payment is at the point of service, and the specifics of any cancellation policies.

During the Consultation

Documentation

Inpatient notes in the medical record are written in a specific fashion to convey a clear, concise, detailed message that other health professionals can share. These messages are commonly displayed in the SOAP note (see Part A of this chapter). As a private practice practitioner, the style in which you document information is up to you. SOAP can be adapted to a longer form if it assists the practitioner with continuity of care. Whether or not the SOAP model is used, an assessment should be created that guides the clinician to ask pertinent questions. Keeping informative, clear notes is important for several reasons:

- Legally, any medical record can be subpoenaed and photocopied.
- Referrals to other health care providers may contain progress notes for resource purposes.

- A detailed, professional summary needs to be sent to the referring physician (see "After the Consultation: Communicating with Professionals" section, later in this chapter).

Determining Weight Goals

Patients who are overweight or obese often feel overwhelmed at the seemingly insurmountable number of pounds they need to lose. Providers need to reassure patients that losing any amount of weight (and keeping it off) can improve health and quality of life.

During the first visit, the clinician will usually observe a degree of discomfort caused by the obesity (eg, the patient might have a hard time moving from a standing to a sitting position). It can be helpful to point this out ("I noticed that it seemed difficult for you to get into a sitting position. Was it?"), both as an empathic gesture and as another measuring point of success when it improves. For some patients, using concrete numbers—such as weight, body mass index (BMI), and waist size—can be helpful in determining goals; for others who are less clear about the role weight plays in health, the more informal quality-of-life assessments can underscore the consequences of excess weight.

All clinical professionals should consider BMI a vital sign. Generally, the higher the BMI, the greater the risk of developing concomitant diseases (9). Therefore, good clinical care includes not only the calculation of BMI, but its inclusion as an indicator of health status in all medical records, letters, and requests. Because it can be difficult to take an accurate height reading given the constraints of private practice, attaching a long tape measure against the wall and having the patient stand against it (in stocking feet) can be useful. BMI can then be calculated from a BMI table.

"Ideal" or "goal" weight, whether assessed by BMI or by other formulas, can provide a quick, rough estimate of ideal goals, but for many clients it will not be realistic. For example, a 65-year-old, sedentary woman who is 5-feet, 2-inches tall and weighs 200 lb, with BMI = 37, weighed 115 pounds (BMI = 21) when she was 25 years old. For the past 10 years, she had been maintaining a weight of 175 lb (BMI = 32). Given these figures, it would be unreasonable for the practitioner to set a weight goal of 115 lb, even if that was the ultimate goal of the client. (The weight would be almost impossible for her to attain, and it would be unnecessary for health improvements.) If she were adamant about a goal of 115 pounds, discuss how small weight changes may result in major improvements in her health profile. Negotiate a shorter-term goal that can be reassessed after it is reached. Trying to dissuade a patient from an ultimate weight goal during the first visit can be unproductive and can put the provider-patient relationship in jeopardy at its earliest stages. However, once a patient has had success in reaching her initial goal and a relationship has been established, a more practical goal can be renegotiated.

Measurement of the waist circumference is also indicative of health risk, independent of BMI (9). However, taking an accurate waist circumference may be inconvenient, because it often means a separate room for disrobing must be available. Clinically, it is most important to measure the waist circumference for individuals with BMI < 35, when the risk from waist size alone is greater.

Although calculating caloric needs through formulas is common, these equations can be burdensome and unnecessary. Given the inaccuracy of the equations and the poor estimates of food intake from diaries (10), it may be more useful to obtain a 24-hour recall or an average daily account. From this information, point out the patterns of consumption that are nonsupportive of weight loss, and help the patient make healthier, low-calorie food choices that are sustainable.

Success is not merely measured by the number of pounds lost. Adopting better eating habits and a consistent exercise plan can prevent further weight gain and improve health. The patient's more positive state of mind, improved shopping habits, normalized blood glucose levels, stable blood pressure levels, and more confident self-image can stem from better management of eating and activity habits, as opposed to greater weight losses. Reducing weight is an additional bonus. Often clinicians forget to communicate this clearly to clients. Defining alternative criteria for clients can help them redefine their own goals.

Nutrition Assessment Interview

The nutrition assessment may be detailed, but the form should be short. It is best to avoid writing or typing a great deal of information during the patient's visit, so that eye contact can be maintained. If possible, leave time between patients to write the assessment after the visit. It is also helpful to leave a space on the form for "miscellaneous" or "other" items—those atypical psychosocial and medical issues that may arise during the session.

During a 60-minute assessment visit, the first half-hour should be spent obtaining information about the patient. The second half becomes an exchange of information, including providing tips to help improve the patient's overall eating habits. The following are tips relevant to private practice (see Figure 2C.1).

General Information. General information can be given to the client before the assessment via mail, e-mail, or in the waiting room. This information includes physician and client contact information, as well as insurance information.

PRIVATE PRACTICE ASSESSMENT NOTE
<u>GENERAL</u>

Name: Jeanine Jones
Address: 425 North Beacon Rd   **Tel. Home:** 123-456-7899
             Talepa, Fla 25325   **Tel. Work:** 123-654-9877
                                          Tel. Cell: _____

Insurance carrier: Guardian
ID # 123-44-5678   **Group #** _____
Name of insured: self

Date of birth: 3/04/45

Referring physician: S. Mason   **Phone #:** 123-777-4200

Job Description: Administrative Assistant, Advertising firm; 9–5

<u>Medical History:</u>
Diabetes, type 2	☐	**Renal disease**	☐
Hyperlipidemia	☐	**Hypertension**	☒
Arthritis	☒	**Other:** high cholesterol	
Gallbladder disease	☐	**Other:** _____	
Liver disease	☐	**Other:** _____	

<u>Medications (incl OTC):</u>
Prinival, 20 mg qd
Calcium on occasion

Last Medical Visit: 2 wks ago

Lives with: Husband + 2 children (15,17)

<u>Family History:</u>
Medical: **Overweight:**
Father: hypertension   Mother: _Yes_____
Mother: type 2 diabetes   Father: _____
                                          Grandmother: _____
                                          Grandfather: _____
                                          Siblings: _____

<u>Social:</u>
Restaurant dining: 2–3 per week   **Business travel:** 0 per year
Take-out: 1 per week   **Vacation:** 1 per year
Favorite foods: Bread   **Alcohol:** on occasion
Foods that are highest risk: Bread, sweets   **Religious/Cultural Beliefs:** n/a
Smoking: no
     # cigarettes: _____

Figure 2C.1. Example of Private-Practice Nutrition Assessment
(continues)

Recent labs: _____ (date)

Cholesterol: 217	**Potassium:** 4.3
LDL-C: 131	**Ast:** _____
HDL-C: 47	**Alt:** _____
Glucose: 106	**Other:** _____
Triglyceride: 175	**Other:** _____
	Other: _____

Height: 64″

Weight History: **Current Weight:**   **BMI:**   **Waist:**

Lowest: 140   224   39   n/a

Highest: 224 (now)

Most usual: 175

Goal weight: to be discussed

DIET HISTORY

Medications: once (fen/phen)	**Weight Watchers:** >3
High-fat, low-carb: twice	**Other:** liquid formula
Low-fat, high-carb: many	**Most successful:** liquid formula

DIETARY RECALL

Breakfast:
½ bagel w/slice cheese
2 coffees w/nonfat milk
Maybe fruit
Wkends: same, w/eggs

After breakfast snacks:
None

Lunch:
Usually sandwich
Regular bread, mustard
Tuna, turkey, ham
Sometimes salad
Drinks: diet soda

After lunch snacks:
Pretzels
Whatever is in office
Sometimes none

Dinner:
Tastes, nibbles while cooking
Veg, lean meat, starch
Drinks water or seltzer
At restaurants: salad, entrée
Taste of someone's dessert
Usually 1–2 glasses wine
Bread basket, no butter

After dinner snacks:
Back and forth to kitchen
Eats anything—standing
Watching television
(est: 500 calories)

Miscellaneous
Hunger sometimes in late afternoon or before dinner

Figure 2C.1. *(Continued)*

(continues)

Assessment:
Although the patient has seen her physician, she is not aware of her risk for diabetes, based on her metabolic syndrome signs (HDL-C, Tg, BP). Glucose shows potential insulin resistance. Dietary recall is vague. Patient admits to regular, unplanned nibbling, particularly when she gets home at night and on weekends. Although she knows what foods are healthy, she admits to last-minute decisions that include high-calorie and fat items. She subscribes to nutritional myths, such as bran muffins being healthier than regular muffins and that pretzels are low-calorie because they are low-fat. Therefore, much of her recall includes phrases such as "I only ate . . . ." Meal replacements and less choice may be helpful, because of their ease. Patient needs to enlist family members for support, if possible. Health will be improved by slow weight loss. Eating behavior at night needs to be addressed.

Plan:
- Meal replacement choices for lunch: OTC formula with one fruit or frozen meal (≤ 300 cal for office or home lunch). In restaurants: salad with grilled fish or chicken, dressing on side, or poached eggs on english muffin with fruit.
- Yogurt + fruit for late afternoon snack or before dinner.
- Dinner: more vegetables, less starch; otherwise, no change for now.
- Night behavior: have children clean up after dinner. Do not go into kitchen, even for tea. Ask husband to assist with any activities in the kitchen after dinner.
- Continue to complete food records; record food intake at the time of eating.
- See me in 1 week. If no weight loss, consider OTC formulas more regularly.

Figure 2C.1. (*Continued*)

Medical Information. It is best to obtain medication information from the primary care physician (see Chapter 3: Clinical Monitoring). The information obtained from the physician may be more accurate than that provided by the patient. In addition, medical guidance can be a vital part of good patient care. If the patient cannot bring medical information to the first visit, make sure you obtain permission from the patient to access the records. Although some clients may know their most abnormal values, it is often the case that they will not know marginal ones.

Social History. Social history includes who the patient lives with, but it also includes outside eating behavior, such as the following items:

- Restaurant dining and take-out. Assess restaurant and take-out eating. If this eating is frequent, suggesting grocery shopping techniques and recipes for home cooking is less important. Focus instead on tips for dining out healthfully. Encourage patients to bring in sets of menus from their favorite dining spots to role-play different ways to order.

- Business travel or entertainment. Is there pressure to eat certain foods? Are there certain trips where overeating is a greater risk? Understanding the different food cultures is important.

Alcohol. Aside from adding calories, alcohol can interact with medications and act as a disinhibitor to overeating. However, unless it is of great risk to health status, be realistic and incorporate occasional drinks into the meal plan.

Smoking. Is smoking used as a substitute for food? Are concerns about weight gain delaying efforts in smoking cessation? Did the client give up smoking recently and replace tobacco with food? Smoking cessation should be encouraged if the client indicates interest. If so, careful dietary monitoring can prevent weight gain during stressful times. Although some people can stop smoking and lose weight at the same time, it is not the norm. It is usually more manageable to change one significant behavior at a time.

Religious or Cultural Beliefs. Clients who observe strict religious or cultural practices often believe they have limited or no food choice. Therefore, it behooves the practitioner to either become familiar with these practices or to ask detailed questions about them so as to better understand the boundaries within which the client must remain. It is important for the practitioner to be accepting of these cultural practices, to evoke an open response to change by the client. In most cases, patients appreciate a dietitian with an understanding of their cultural practices. With today's greater recognition and respect for alternative medicine, health professionals and educators have a responsibility to learn about and to accept cultural beliefs that may seem incongruent with their own, so long as the patient is not harmed (11,12).

Psychosocial Issues. One of the most challenging aspects of counseling is getting a client to identify, and then to overcome, barriers to change (2). It is common for clients to be knowledgeable about diets and skilled at giving advice to others but to be unable to apply this knowledge in their own lives. At the assessment, it can be helpful to communicate this to the client and to explain that experimentation is important for long-term success of any diet. Encourage clients to write down all their efforts and to measure them as supportive or not supportive. Not only does this help them to create their own toolbox, but it will help the provider to tailor certain tools in follow-up sessions.

Usual Diet

A patient's dietary recall is pivotal in determining the type of plan that will be recommended. Some clinicians like to use a 24-hour recall, but the past 24 hours could have reflected the eating style of someone who anticipated being asked such questions and, therefore, consumed food while on "their best behavior" (10,13). For others, the day before a consultation with a nutritionist could resemble a "Last Supper," where significant overeating occurs in anticipation of a period of severe restriction. Although the most commonly used dietary questionnaire is the food frequency questionnaire, this also has its weaknesses: the list of specific foods is not culturally specific, nor does it assess current energy intake (10). Therefore, obtaining information about usual dietary practices may be useful in helping the patient to create a more realistic next step. But it takes some skill to elicit the information.

Dealing With Imperfection.   The patient has to trust the provider enough to be able to describe overeating episodes in some detail. Most people will label eating habits and food choices as either "good" or "bad." In order to suggest guidelines for the future, *all* habits of the past need to be addressed. If the person sitting in front of you has been a hummingbird of diets, jumping from one to another on a regular basis, it may be important to pay close attention to what constitutes "good" days. These days may have produced a weight loss, but were probably too strict and unrealistic. It is essential to listen to the detail of a "bad" day, because these probably include foods that the patient craves or enjoys but perhaps withholds when "on a diet" and binges on when "off." When devising a meal plan for this type of patient, be sure to include some of the so-called "bad" foods, to prevent relapse and to help develop a realistic rather than punitive approach.

Open-ended Questions.   Obtaining a listing of daily foods can be waitress-like and tedious; yet there is much to be learned from such a listing, especially if using open-ended questions. For example, it is best to refrain from asking, "Do you use dressing on your salad?" because most people will think they should answer that question with a "No." The question, "What kind of dressing do you like on your salad?" will prompt a more realistic response that may segue to further discussion (14). This kind of questioning can also elicit more honest behavioral habits, such as eating while watching TV, driving a car, or standing in front of the refrigerator (see Practical Applications section of Chapter 4: Behavioral Treatment).

Reviewing the Dietary Record.   Some clinicians have their patients fill out a detailed food record before their first consultation. The form is sent to the patient in preparation for the first visit. Although this procedure may save time during the interview, asking these questions in person gives the clinician the opportunity to ask additional pertinent questions, as well as to see the patient's facial expressions. Assessing clients in person as they recall the food intake—whether they falter as they speak about certain eating events or what they might forget and suddenly remember—can be invaluable information that could not be observed in a written form.

The private practice provider has to be prepared for the patient who does not keep food records. Although in private practice it is difficult to make a food diary a requirement, a patient's lack of commitment to write down what he or she eats triggers concerns about a willingness to carefully review habits and make necessary changes. Food diaries should be encouraged and are especially helpful for those who eat for reasons other than physical hunger (eg, stress or boredom). Many overweight patients eat unconsciously, at their desks, in their cars, and in front of TV sets or computer monitors. Keeping food records helps to increase the awareness of these eating episodes (10).

After the Consultation: Communicating With Professionals

Before consulting with a patient, it is helpful to speak with his or her physician (to obtain lab reports and background information). Although this contact is not always possible, it is critical to send a note to the physician (or other referral source) after the meeting, outlining the assessment of the patient's nutritional status and the treatment plan. This summary report will not only shed light on the nutritional aspects of the patient's health status that the doctor may or may not have been aware of, but it also casts you as an invaluable resource who holds an important place in the health care team. Professionally written reports will help ensure that you will receive future needed lab or medical reports (7,8). In all cases, professional communication needs to be ethical and responsible, with the goal being to transfer clear information that is accurate. Objectivity is essential, and conciseness is imperative.

Communication can be established by sending a letter that briefly describes your visit with the patient. A template of a form letter will make it easier to write (8). This form could be as simple as containing the patient's name, height and weight, date of birth, diagnosis, pertinent lab reports, medications taken, diet history, and your impression. A space can also be provided for additional comments (eg, the patient's family does not appear to be supportive or weekly follow-ups have been scheduled). Some clinicians prefer to send a standard cover letter and a copy of the assessment sheet used during the initial consultation. A condensed follow-up report can then be sent when necessary.

Final Note

As Dittoe states (15), the nutrition interview could become a "major turning point in clients' lives," by helping them to understand their problems and personal issues more clearly. This association could help them "get to the root of many of their long-standing behaviors and thoughts that have been complicating their lives for years" (15). To truly help clients, providers need to expand their scope of knowledge beyond the realm of clinical dietetics (see Chapter 4: Behavioral Treatment). The greatest quality the practitioner can possess is empathy. By understanding a client's daily living situation, even subtle changes could produce major long-term benefits.

References

1. Coulston AM, Feenedy MJ, Hoolihan L. The challenge to customize. *J Am Diet Assoc.* 2003;103:443–444.
2. Molaison EF. Stages of change in clinical nutrition practice. *Nutr Clin Care.* 2002;5:251–257.
3. Dalton CC, Gottlieb LN. The concept of readiness to change. *J Adv Nurs.* 2003;42:108–117.
4. Steptoe A, Perkins-Porras L, McKay C, Rink E, Hilton S, Cappuccio FP. Behavioural counselling to increase consumption of fruit and vegetables in low income adults: randomised trial. *BMJ.* 2003;326:855– 961.
5. Chernoff R, ed. *Communicating as Professionals.* 2nd ed. Chicago, Ill: American Dietetic Association; 1994.
6. Israel D, Moores S, eds. *Beyond Nutrition Counseling.* Chicago, Ill: American Dietetic Association; 1996.
7. Cummings S, Parham ES, Strain GW. Position of the American Dietetic Association: weight management. *J Am Diet Assoc.* 2002;102:1145–1155.
8. Kuppersmith NC, Wheeler SF. Communication between family physicians and registered dietitians in the outpatient setting. *J Am Diet Assoc.* 2002;102:1756–1763.
9. National Heart, Lung, and Blood Institute, National Institutes of Health. *Clinical Guidelines on the Identification, Evaluation, and Treatment of Overweight and Obesity in Adults.* Bethesda, Md: National Institutes of Health; 2002. NIH Publication No. 98-4083.
10. Johnson RK. Dietary intake—how do we measure what people are really eating? *Obes Res.* 2002;10(Suppl 1):63S–68S.
11. Mercer SL, Green LW, Rosenthal AC, Husten CG, Khan LK, Dietz WH. Possible lessons from the tobacco experience for obesity control. *Am J Clin Nutr.* 2003;77:1073S–1082S.
12. Sue WD, Sue D. *Counseling the Culturally Different: Theory and Practice.* 3rd ed. New York, NY: John Wiley & Sons; 1999.
13. Engelman K, Mattes RD. Insignificant data cannot yield statistically significant conclusions. *Arch Intern Med.* 2003;163:851–855.

14. Rosal MC, Ebbeling CB, Lofgren I, Ockene JK, Ockene IS, Hebert JR. Facilitating dietary change: the patient-centered counseling model. *J Am Diet Assoc.* 2001;101:332–341.
15. Dittoe AB. Teaching developmental skills when counseling adults. In: Helm KK, Klawitter B, eds. *Nutrition Therapy: Advanced Counseling Skills.* Lake Dallas, Tex: Helm Seminars; 1995:101–112.

Chapter 3
Clinical Monitoring

PART A. Overview

F. Xavier Pi-Sunyer, MD, MPH

Importance of Monitoring Symptoms During Weight Loss

Among clinicians who care for obese patients, it is well known that obesity increases the risk of various medical conditions and that weight loss typically improves these conditions. It is also true, however, that complications can occur, and some diseases may worsen with weight loss (1). Thus, all health professionals should be aware of conditions associated with obesity and of possible concomitant risks that can occur during weight loss. This section defines some of the typical physiological changes that can occur during weight loss and suggests how the nonphysician and physician can work as a team to provide optimal clinical monitoring during weight loss.

Working With a Physician

Although it seems obvious to suggest establishing a relationship with the physician, all too often this step is overlooked. Without it, treatment can be significantly hampered. Before initiating any treatment plan for weight loss, it is best for the clinician to receive, from the client's physician, a copy of the most recent physical, including a thorough medical history, medications currently being used (including those that are associated with weight gain), an EKG interpretation, and a complete laboratory test (2). This medical assessment then becomes the blueprint for the appropriate pattern of follow-up. (If the physician has not indicated a schedule for medical follow-up, it is important to request it.) This plan should be reviewed with the patient at the initial and follow-up visits, to underscore the importance of medical follow-up. Follow-up is particularly important for patients taking medications that are likely to be affected by modest weight loss (eg, oral hypoglycemics or antihypertensives). If the patient sees the nonphysician first, it is important for this clinician to refer the patient back to the primary care physician for a full workup before starting any diet that suggests anything other than modest changes.

There are many scenarios in which the physician–clinical specialist relationship is crucial to appropriate care of the patient. Whether or not the physician and the weight management clinician work in the same office or even know each other, it is important that they work as a team. For example, for a patient who has diabetes and is on multiple medications, it is necessary to have information about baseline lab values (including the EKG) and a recent review of systems, in order to set a protocol strategy that prevents hypoglycemia when the lower-calorie prescription is being followed. This protocol should entail the frequency of assessing adjustments in diabetes medications as the patient loses weight. Once this protocol is established by the physician, each member of the team should be able to fulfill his or her responsibilities and to act in concert with the others to reduce complications. If a patient is on blood pressure medication, how often does the blood pressure need to be reevaluated in order to prevent hypotension? What are the signs for the nonphysician that it would be appropriate to refer the patient back to the primary care physician sooner?

Selected Conditions That Require Monitoring

Heart Disease

People with already existing heart disease should have the heart assessed and any medications noted before beginning a diet for weight loss. Although these patients generally experience an improvement of their heart disease with weight loss, they should be monitored regularly. Therefore, if the patient has not had an EKG recently, the clinician should refer back to the physician for a baseline, and then request a follow-up protocol. During the acute weight-loss phase, many complications can arise. Patients often have a significant diuresis and/or they lose weight too quickly. Abnormalities, arrhythmias, or congestive heart failure are quite common and often go undetected until there is a problem during the weight-loss process. Replacement of adequate sodium, potassium, and magnesium may be important, particularly during the initial diuresis. Electrolyte abnormalities can lead to cardiac arrhythmias that are best prevented by adequate attention to micronutrient balance. In the short or long term, weight loss can cause a catabolic state in the heart, often manifested by changes in the QT interval (3). This may require that the practitioner stop or modify the hypocaloric diet. An electrocardiogram at intervals during the diet (timed according to the severity of the caloric deficit and the cardiac status of the patient) is an important monitoring requirement. Again, the team is critical here. How often should the patient see the primary care physician or, in this case, the cardiologist? Should the rate of weight loss be more conservative? The same consideration should be given to abnormal lab values, hyperlipidemia, or sleep apnea (4). Documentation of telephone conversations and meetings about the patient should be updated in the chart.

Gallbladder Disease

Another common complication is gallbladder disease. Gallstones often form or the disease becomes symptomatic during a weight-loss attempt (5). This is because of a high supersaturation of bile with cholesterol and a poor contraction of the gallbladder. There are some preventive measures, as discussed in Part B of this chapter, but the clinical provider needs to know what signs might be indicative of the disease, so that referral back to the physician is done in a timely manner, to prevent more severe complications.

Initiating Physical Activity

Exercise is important during weight loss and imperative for weight-loss maintenance (2). Physical activity needs to be initiated or increased and then maintained to help prevent the regain of weight that is so common among dieters (see Part A of Chapter 9: Weight-Loss Maintenance). Before an exercise regimen is started, it is necessary (1) to check for foot and orthopedic problems, (2) to make sure there is no neuropathy, and (3) to assess the condition of the heart. Although full cardiac testing does not need to be done on everyone, it is a good idea for those with a history of coronary heart disease, cardiac failure, or dyslipidemia. Again, when weight management experts— whether dietitians, exercise physiologists, or psychotherapists—suggest physical activity, they must first ask the physician for patient clearance (or follow guidelines in Part B of Chapter 6: Physical Activity).

Constipation

Some patients develop constipation or diarrhea during their diet. These conditions are not usually serious and generally disappear with time. However, persistent symptoms should be appropriately monitored and the patient should be referred back to the physician.

Psychiatric Status

An awareness of the psychiatric status of the patient is also required, with frequent monitoring. Although most obese patients will experience mood improvements, some will become more depressed with both the deprivation that they experience from a reduction of their favorite foods and the change in body size. An alert health professional will look for telltale signs (eg, sleep disturbance, sadness, hopelessness, inability to experience pleasure) of increased depression and refer appropriately.

Conclusion

Weight loss causes major pathophysiological changes in the body, most of which are positive. Nonetheless, the practitioner needs to be aware of possible adverse side effects and should try to prevent them through team care. A solid medical evaluation before weight loss, from which a follow-up protocol is created, will significantly reduce the chance of complications during the weight-loss phase. No matter what the initial protocol, it behooves the provider to refer back to the primary care physician any time there is even a slight concern about a patient's symptoms. These communications—whether by telephone, letter, or part of a patient's chart—are key in assessing a patient's health status throughout weight loss and into weight maintenance. Without them, care can be disjointed and health compromised. By contrast, a united team effort provides the patient with the best care possible and increases the likelihood of a healthy and successful outcome.

References

1. Pi-Sunyer FX. Medical hazards of obesity. *Ann Intern Med*. 1993;119:655–660.
2. National Institutes of Health. Clinical guidelines on the identification, evaluation, and treatment of overweight and obesity in adults—the evidence report. *Obes Res*. 1998;6(Suppl 2):S51–S209.
3. Van Itallie TB, Yang MU. Cardiac dysfunction in obese dieters: a potentially lethal complication of rapid, massive weight loss. *Am J Clin Nutr*. 1984; 39:695–702.
4. Pi-Sunyer FX. A review of long-term studies evaluating the efficacy of weight loss in ameliorating disorders associated with obesity. *Clin Ther*. 1996;18: 1006–1035.
5. Heshka S, Spitz A, Nunez C, Fittante AM, Heymsfield SB, Pi-Sunyer FX. Obesity and risk of gallstone development on a 1200 kcal/d (5025 Kj/d) regular food diet. *Int J Obes Relat Metab Disord*. 1996;20:450–454.

PART B. Practical Applications

Cathy A. Nonas, MS, RD, CDE

Unlike almost any other disease, obesity is one in which there are no set guidelines for monitoring a patient. The fundamental metric of relative weight, body mass index (BMI), is seldom documented. In a study of 10,000 physicians, more than 50% did not discuss weight with a patient, even when the patient was obese (1). Most primary physicians treat the concomitant risks, such as hypertension, diabetes, and dyslipidemia, rather than the obesity itself. This is extremely unfortunate, given that obese individuals have a 50% to 100% increased risk of death from all causes, compared with normal-weight individuals (Figure 3B.1) (2).

On referral, even broad-based goals, such as "lose 5% to 10% of weight and then return to my office for reevaluation," are infrequent. Detailed protocols, such as "lose 1 to 2 pounds per week and return for electrolyte and blood pressure readings after every 10-pound weight loss," are rarely suggested. More often, there is no physician referral, only a patient's desire to lose weight. But to treat the patient appropriately during weight

Health Risks:	Compared to BMI at:	Body Mass Index 26 27 28 29 30 31 32 33 34 35
Death/All Causes	< 19	60% 110% 120%
Death/Heart Diseases	< 19	210% 360% 480%
Death/Cancer	< 19	80% 110%
Type II Diabetes	22–23	1,480% 2,660% 3,930% 5,300%
High Blood Pressure	< 23	180% 260% 350%
Degenerative Arthritis	< 25	400%
Gallstones	< 24	150% 270%
Neural Birth Defects	19–27	90%

Figure 3B.1.   Relative Increase in Risk by BMI
Adapted with permission from Centers for Obesity Research and Education. Weighing the Risks (unpublished handout). Denver, Colo: Centers for Obesity Research and Education.

loss, two clinicians—the physician and the nonphysician provider—must become a team. A comprehensive obesity assessment describes an appropriate diet and lifestyle change on the basis of a patient's readiness and health status (see Chapter 2: Assessment). Once the diet (weight loss) begins, these same issues need to be monitored. The difference is that the health status is *constantly changing* and must be monitored as well. The dietetics professional, the exercise physiologist, or the counselor may be the only source of support for the patient during weight loss. Therefore, case management becomes the responsibility of the provider who sees the patient most frequently. The American Dietetic Association's (ADA) position on weight management allows for this fact: "The dietitian can play a pivotal role in modifying weight status by helping to formulate reasonable goals which can be met and sustained with a healthy eating approach . . . Any changes in dietary intake and exercise patterns which decrease caloric intake below energy expenditure will result in weight loss, but it is the responsibility of the dietitian to make sure the changes recommended are directed toward improved physiological and psychological health" (3).

This chapter attempts to help the nonphysician case manage appropriately by explaining the most common diseases associated with obesity and the "team protocol" that may be created.

The Team

Good clinical care for obesity demands a team approach, even though the "team" may not always be within the same site. It is often the responsibility of the nonphysician to design that team, as well as to serve as the case manager. The physician does the medical oversight, but the nonphysician is the one to prompt patients to return to their physician. In most cases, the patient's comorbidities are improved with weight loss, and the physician visits become less frequent. The goal for obesity treatment is to reduce excess body fat and the comorbidities associated with obesity. However, the diabetes paradigm shows that duration of disease and lack of control of concomitant complications may lead to worsening of the disease (4). It is the same with obesity (5). Therefore, a health care professional who is seeing the patient for weight loss has to remain aware of the risks inherent during weight loss and the best way to triage these problems.

Monitoring weight occurs in two phases: acute and chronic. These phases seesaw. When a patient is beginning to lose weight, he or she is in the acute phase; after a couple of months, as weight loss slows, the patient is in the chronic stage. If the patient regains significant amounts of weight over time, then a new weight-loss regimen may be warranted and the patient returns to the acute stage.

Box 3B.1. Some Acute Reasons to Refer to the Physician

- Arrhythmia, chest pain complaints
- Upper right quadrant pain (gallbladder)
- Sudden dizziness, headaches, or cognitive changes
- Hyperuricemia, gouty inflammations, and joint pain
- Bowels—changes to diarrhea or constipation for more than a couple of days
- Skin color—may change to dull yellow or greenish tinge
- Sudden depression
- Rapid weight loss
- Edema
- Lower extremities have skin breaks that are not healing

Excess fat causes metabolic changes, such as gallbladder disease, dyslipidemia, insulin resistance, hypertension, polycystic ovarian syndrome, coronary artery disease, and diabetes mellitus. It also causes physical changes, such as sleep apnea, cardiac structural changes, cellulitis, and osteoarthritis. Therefore, changing the level of body fat will alter the diseases associated with excess fat. In general, the more obese the patient, the more numerous the complications. Likewise, associated risks tend to manifest themselves more frequently in people older than 40 years (6).

But any change in weight status may increase risks. If there is a higher risk of death and disease due to an increase in weight, then the additional stress of changing weight may cause morbidities to worsen. By understanding some of the risks that may occur, the clinician can refer the patient back to the physician at appropriate times, which reduces risks for the patient. If the patient becomes symptomatic (eg, is lightheaded or has leg cramps) it is important to document it, refer the patient to the primary physician, and then obtain feedback from the physician. Is the patient exhibiting symptoms that are related to diet or weight loss? If so, what dietary changes are made?

Fat Distribution Changes the Risk Profile

Gynoid (Lower-Body) Obesity

Obesity alone increases health risk. However, an obese person whose fat is distributed in the lower body (buttocks and thigh) experiences fewer comorbidities than the one who has a more android, or upper body, obesity (stomach and waist). Even among severely obese patients with BMIs as high as 50 or 60, major complaints may consist solely of osteoarthritis. The

---

Box 3B.2. Some "Obesity Diseases" During Weight Loss

- Diabetes—adjust medications as per daily blood sugars.
- Hypertension—evaluate medications after 5% weight loss or as indicated by patient's symptoms.
- Lipids—metabolic syndrome, hyperlipidemia, and dyslipidemia, if weight related, will change within the first 3 to 6 weeks.
- Arthritis—individual improvement seen throughout weight loss.
- Fatty liver—should be improved within first 6 weeks.
- Insulin resistance—does not need to be monitored. Will improve in most cases as a result of weight loss.

---

lower-body obesity (extremely large hips and thighs, edematous ankles) is less likely to be associated with hypertension, diabetes, or dyslipidemia. Pressure from overweight is significant, particularly in the knees. It is extremely painful to sit and stand up. Chairs are usually too narrow to fit the width of the hips once the patient sits down. Many need to walk with a cane. Weight loss, even small amounts, has a rapid effect, reducing pain at least a little and making it easier for the patient to move.

Team Protocol.   Some arthritis medications can increase weight, so it is helpful to ask the patient if there was a weight change since taking the medication. A patient such as this, who exhibits no other comorbidities but osteoarthritis, may need less monitoring by a physician during weight loss, as long as all the baseline evaluations have been performed and the physician agrees.

Android (Upper-Body) Obesity

As described in Chapter 2: Assessment, measurement of waist circumference is not indicated among those with BMI ≥ 35 because class II obesity and extreme obesity are extremely dangerous no matter how fat is distributed. For individuals with BMIs between 30 and 35, waist circumference should be measured. However, the risks inherent in class I obesity itself are significant enough to monitor the patient frequently and aggressively to try to prevent further risk. For patients with a BMI < 30, it is important to measure waist circumference because the risk of disease is greater if waist circumference is >100 cm (5), although the consequences of abdominal fat may not be the same for all ethnic groups (7). Decisions about how aggressively to test for other risk factors, as well as the nature of the weight-loss regimen will be affected by information about waist circumference.

Team Protocol. This is where the clinical professional can help with triaging the patient. Waist circumference is one measurement that can help give information on the risk for disease or how often the patient might have to be monitored. The team should be more aggressive about weight loss and monitoring those with higher waist circumferences. Therefore, if the clinician is uncomfortable with measuring the waist, a note should be written to the physician suggesting that the physician (or the patient) measure the waist periodically to assess risk during weight loss. Reductions in waist circumference are a simple way to document success and improved health.

Rate of Weight Loss

During the first 2 weeks of a weight-loss diet, the patient will lose water, both from the decrease in sodium consumption and from the mobilization of glycogen. Glycogen has water molecules attached to it, so both carbohydrate stores and water are lost in the process. Although there are some patients, usually women, who may not diurese as much as expected, most will have their largest weight losses in these first 2 weeks. After this diuresis, the rate of weight loss should be considerably slower. A pound of weight is part lean, part fat tissue, and as a person loses weight, the goal is for that pound to be at least 75% fat, 25% lean (8,9). Conveniently, this is equal to approximately 3,200 to 3,500 kcal, depending on the exact ratio of fat-to-lean. If someone were to lose 1 pound of only fat, then the pound would be equal to approximately 4,200 kcal. Because of the differences in the energy attributed to protein and fat, the speed at which someone loses weight may be indicative of additional stress on the heart tissue (protein) (10,11). Restricting the rate of weight loss after diuresis to either 1 to 2 lb per week or 1% of initial weight will help ensure that a pound of weight lost contains mostly fat (5).

Team Protocol. If diuresis is >10 lb in the first week, call the referring physician for guidance. If the patient loses more than 1% of weight per week for 3 consecutive weeks after diuresis is complete, call the physician and increase the number of calories by 200-kcal/day increments.

Monitoring Risks During Weight Loss

Hypoglycemia

If a patient with type 2 diabetes takes medication to control blood sugar, a very common side effect in the first month is hypoglycemia. If the patient is tightly controlled, weight loss, without a compensatory adjustment in diabetes medication, will result in low blood sugar, regardless of the dietary guidelines. Often a clinical team does not consider this fact, although it is well known that weight loss causes the blood sugars to reduce and, sometimes, to plummet. Many clinicians suggest that a patient eat a couple of graham crackers if he or she experiences hypoglycemic symptoms. Prescribing extra food for an obese patient to avoid hypoglycemia is counterproductive and inappropriate. Instead, ask the physician to lower the medication, which gives you the option to decrease the food even more. Likewise, waiting until the patient complains about hypoglycemia can be dangerous because hypoglycemia can result in imbalance, vomiting, severe headaches, and unconsciousness. If the patient is on diabetes medication and does not monitor blood sugars, the focus should be on getting the patient to begin monitoring.

Team Protocol.   Discuss hypoglycemia potential with the patient and with the physician. Establish a range for blood sugar and identify the point at which the patient should contact the physician for further medication adjustment.

Hypokalemia

During the first few weeks of weight loss, as the body diureses and weight loss is most rapid, side effects may occur. These include dehydration, electrolyte abnormalities, and cardiac arrhythmias. Although potassium is usually not a problem during this time, it is important to monitor this electrolyte during the first month, in particular. A very restrictive diet for 1 or 2 weeks that causes a large diuresis may result in hypokalemia, particularly in those whose potassium is initially borderline normal. Therefore, it is helpful to monitor serum potassium during the diuresis stage. What is the baseline serum potassium? Is it low normal (eg, 3.9 mEq/dL) or is it midrange (eg, 4.5 mEq/dL)? The baseline value may help the physician decide whether to supplement the diet. Are serum potassium values dropping, even within normal range during weight loss (eg, from 4.5 to 3.9 mEq/dL)? From this information, the physician may want to supplement.

Team Protocol.   If the patient is on a diuretic, ask the physician if lowering the dose or stopping the diuretic altogether is appropriate, particularly when the patient is following a very-low-calorie diet, in which the diuresis might be significant. If the patient's serum potassium is low normal (eg, 3.9 mEq/dL), should he or she be prescribed 20 mEq of potassium supplement? If the serum potassium is falling during weight loss, should the patient be prescribed 20 mEq of potassium supplement as a preventive measure to guard against hypokalemia? When should the nonphysician send the patient to the lab for follow-up testing?

Cellulitis

Cellulitis is caused by reduced skin integrity. The body's surface area is enlarged, and the heart cannot pump enough blood to all parts of the body, particularly the legs. Skin tissue begins to break down and cellulitis results. If a patient complains about any unusual leg pain, one thing to ask is whether they have extreme redness, any change in temperature, or any sores.

Team Protocol. If either the patient or you suspects cellulitis, have the patient contact the physician immediately for antibiotics.

Hyperuricemia

Obesity, particularly upper-body obesity, is associated with higher uric acid levels (12). Red wine and purines are known to aggravate uric acid levels (13), but a very-low-calorie or very-low-carbohydrate diet can also cause levels to increase (14,15). Ketone bodies, products of fat oxidation while a patient is on a very-low-carbohydrate diet, compete with urate for tubular reabsorption in the kidney. This causes an increase in uric acid levels. Adding carbohydrates to the diet and slowing the rate of weight loss will usually reduce the risks.

Team Protocol. If the patient has had a history of gout or if the patient has an abnormally high uric acid, monitor serum bloods during the first 6 weeks of weight loss in order to reduce risk.

Insulin Resistance

Insulin resistance is a disorder that occurs when tissues become less responsive to the action of normal amounts of insulin. Insulin production in the pancreas is then increased, to compensate for this insensitivity. Insulin resistance commonly occurs with obesity, particularly in abdominal obesity. The fat cells are larger in the abdominal area, and the normal flow of fatty acids to the liver becomes faster. Insulin is secreted by the beta cells of the pancreas, most of which are sent through the portal vein to the liver for processing. When the fat distribution is in the lower body, there is less insensitivity.

Weight loss itself will improve insulin resistance—no matter what the diet. Increased pancreatic insulin secretion in obesity is directly related to increased body weight. Therefore, decreasing the weight decreases the insulin resistance. The Diabetes Prevention Program, a national, randomized, clinical trial sponsored by the National Institutes of Health (NIH), compared incidence of conversion to type 2 diabetes in adults with glucose intolerance (16). The study compared three arms: control, drug, and lifestyle. The drug intervention was metformin, which decreases hepatic glucose production and improves insulin sensitivity by increasing peripheral glucose use. In some studies, it has also resulted in weight loss. The lifestyle arm of the study included a low-fat diet, 150 minutes of activity each week, and 7% weight loss. Lifestyle reduced the risk of converting to diabetes by 58%, as compared to metformin, which reduced risk by 31%.

Team Protocol.   If a very rigid diet is attempted with someone who may be insulin resistant with or without impaired glucose tolerance, a baseline EKG, fasting glucose, and lipid levels help to identify any associated risk factors. Otherwise, weight loss is the appropriate treatment, with follow-up labs to monitor lipids, glucose, and electrolytes.

Sleep Apnea

Obstructive sleep apnea is characterized by multiple, brief interruptions of breathing during sleep despite continued inspiratory effort. Sleep apnea can have a variety of cardiovascular and psychosocial consequences, inclding hypertension, impaired quality of life, and motor vehicle accidents (17). Obesity, particularly upper-body obesity, is a strong risk factor for sleep apnea (18). Obesity can lead to a narrowing in the upper airway structure, due to an accumulation of subcutaneous or periluminal fat deposits on the pharynx or fatty infiltration around the neck. Weight loss is associated with improvements in the sleep apnea, although the results are variable (19). Therefore, the physician should evaluate the level of risk, and the nonphysician who suspects sleep apnea should refer back to the physician for a rule-out. A sleep study can diagnose the severity of the apnea, and, if necessary, continuous positive airway pressure (CPAP) (a breathing apparatus used during sleep) can be prescribed.

> *Example:* A patient, SH, has had three visits. He has a visibly thick neck—thicker than most overweight men. At the first visit, he indicated that he had not been diagnosed with sleep apnea. Over time, he has reported that he sleeps well, but occasionally he complains of being tired in the mornings and sometimes he finds himself nodding off at boring meetings or in front of the television. Hypoglycemia was ruled out in the first visit. You ask him if he snores. "Yes," he says; his wife always complains about it. (About 16% of people who snore habitually have sleep apnea, with more than 30 respiratory episodes per night) (18). Has his physician ruled out sleep apnea?

> *Team Protocol.*   If the signs of sleep apnea (snoring, gasping, or choking during sleep) are apparent, send the patient back to the physician with a

note asking to rule out this possibility. Furthermore, get a response from the physician to ensure that weight loss will not add further risk to his cardiac status. However, if a patient knows that he has sleep apnea but is noncompliant with CPAP, the clinician would want to make the physician aware of it.

The Heart

Overweight and obesity are associated with a number of cardiac abnormalities, including arrhythmias, sudden death, and congestive heart failure (20–23). Given that the function of the heart is to pump blood throughout the body, a larger body requires the heart to work harder in order to pump blood to all its parts. There is expanded lean mass and skin, as well as increased fat tissue, which results in higher oxidative needs. Pumping of the blood is work performed mostly by the left ventricle, and in obese people the left ventricular area is often enlarged compared with that of controls. However, the increase in ventricular mass is in direct response to an increase in BMI (23) and helps to compensate for the increased cardiac output. Stroke volume is increased, but heart rate and blood pressure tend to remain within normal range (albeit high normal) until much later in cardiac disease. Therefore, if the patient is both obese and hypertensive, the amount of cardiac work is even more significant. Once the heart can no longer adapt to volume overload (it cannot compensate enough for the increased need of an increased body size), the heart begins to fail. Both filling and pumping are reduced.

Arrhythmia

An arrhythmia is a change in the regular beat of the heart. The heart may seem to skip a beat or beat irregularly or very fast or very slowly. When you take the pulse rate, you can feel the unevenness of the beat. Not everyone measures blood pressure and heart rate, nor should they. Although arrhythmias are not the norm, they are not uncommon. Therefore, it is good clinical practice between the physician and the nonphysician to set up a protocol to monitor the patient's heart rate and blood pressure on a regular basis. This is a safety rule for all patients, because anyone who is obese and losing weight is at risk. Another good practice is to ask for a baseline EKG and periodic EKGs. Frequently, when a patient has a complaint and an EKG is done, there is no baseline EKG to use for comparison. If it is an abnormal EKG, it might have been an abnormality that was stable and nonthreatening, but if no one knows, the weight-loss diet becomes the culprit and is discontinued.

Team Protocol.   Although weight loss usually improves cardiovascular disease, there are obese individuals whose hearts have been irreparably damaged and for whom the stressors of weight loss will be too great (24,25). Therefore, it is imperative that there be clear communication between physician and clinician before putting a patient on a weight-loss diet. The protocol should include a baseline EKG, labs, and physician approval for the specific diet, as well as a schedule as to who monitors heart rate and how often it is done. Depending on the dietary restriction and the patient's present health profile, follow-up to the physician could be more frequent initially and then every 2 months. Physician visits should include EKGs periodically, as well as, at a minimum, after every 50 lb of weight loss.

Lipoprotein Metabolism

As adults and children become more overweight, lipids rise. Obesity and weight gain are associated with increased serum cholesterol, LDL-C, and triglycerides, as well as with decreased HDL-C. The pattern of fat distribution also has a direct relationship with lipid levels, independent of weight. Obesity and weight gain, as well as lifestyle change, are key to improving the lipoprotein metabolism. In fact, therapeutic lifestyle change is considered a treatment for metabolic syndrome, a constellation of factors that are used to define risk of cardiovascular disease.

Example: Patient HS weighs 340 lb, with a BMI of 54. He and his physician are relieved that he is in relatively good health. His total cholesterol is 128. His glucose is within normal limits. No, he did not have an EKG. Maybe he'll get one on his next physician visit.

It is one of the quirks of obesity that severely obese people do not always exhibit high plasma cholesterol levels. As a matter of fact, sometimes the blood cholesterol level is extremely low. Does that mean that the obese person is free of coronary artery risk? No. It simply means that serum cholesterol is not the only determinant of an unhealthy heart.

The clinician asks HS what his HDL-C is. He does not know, but he says that his total cholesterol is so low that his physician told him it did not matter. You ask the same thing about his triglycerides, and he gives you the same answer. Why does HS want to lose weight? "I'm too fat," he says. "I should lose weight." HS should—but is this enough of an incentive for him to do so? If he thinks he is perfectly healthy and that there are no health risks to improve with a healthier lifestyle, what is his motivation? "Well, I am glad you are here," you respond.

"And if it's all right with you, I'm going to call your doctor to get a copy of your latest blood work."

The clinician would like the diet to improve the health profile. But sometimes the subtle shifts in results may be more remarkable to the expert in weight management than to the patient. Therefore, it is part of the clinician's job to enlighten patients enough so that when there is improvement, it is one more success, one more demonstration of improved self-care, one extra buffer against heart disease and sudden death.

Team Protocol. A patient is usually referred for blood tests after the physician visit, with the physician evaluating results afterward. Then, unless the blood tests indicate a serious condition in need of immediate treatment, it is not uncommon for nothing more to be done until the next physician visit. This visit, if scheduled at all, may not happen for 6 months or more. Therefore, if total cholesterol is >250 mg/dL, a note should be written by the clinician to the referring physician suggesting the patient schedule a follow-up visit with him or her after 6 weeks of weight loss. Furthermore, if total cholesterol or triglycerides are >300 mg/dL, then the letter should indicate that diet and/or weight loss may not reduce the lipids enough. If a patient meets the Third Report of the National Cholesterol Education Program (NCEP) Expert Panel on Detection, Evaluation, and Treatment of High Blood Cholesterol in Adults (Adult Treatment Panel III [ATP III]) guidelines for pharmacotherapy, this should be noted (26), and the physician queried as to when he or she wants to reevaluate the patient.

Metabolic Syndrome

If HS has low HDL-C (38 mg/dL) with a fasting glucose of 112 and no symptoms, most clinicians would consider him to be in relatively good health. This is not necessarily the case. Add one more risk factor, such as serum triglycerides that are 175 mg/dL, and you have a patient who has metabolic syndrome (27) and is at risk for ischemic heart disease (Box 3B.3). Each risk factor can be important, and together they give clinicians a better picture of the patient's health status, thereby helping to indicate more appropriate treatment options. The first line of treatment for metabolic syndrome is lifestyle change.

A low HDL-C and borderline triglycerides would be indicative of LDL-C particles that were small and atherogenic, no matter what the total LDL-C was. If no one is monitoring HS, it is very possible that his health will worsen significantly, not improve.

> **Box 3B.3. Risk factors for Metabolic Syndrome**
>
> Patient must have 3 out of the following 5 risk factors:
>
> - Abdominal obesity (waist circumference ≥35 inches in women, ≥40 inches in men)
> - Fasting triglycerides ≥150 mg/dL
> - HDL-C <40 mg/dL in men; <50 mg/dL in women
> - Raised blood pressure (without diagnosis of hypertension ≥130/85)
> - Fasting serum glucose ≥110 mg/dL

Team Protocol. Usually lipids improve during weight loss. However, there is a short-term dip in HDL-C, and sometimes, because of the lipoprotein turnover, there is a short-term increase in serum cholesterol. A lipoprotein profile (HDL-C, total cholesterol, LDL-C, and triglycerides) should be assessed regularly, according to a schedule set up by the physician (every 6 to 8 weeks is usual). Anyone who has dyslipidemia should also have a baseline EKG and regular EKG follow-ups.

Blood Pressure

There are approximately 50 million adults in the United States who have hypertension, classified as a blood pressure reading of 140/90 mm Hg (28). More than 38 million American adults are prehypertensive, with blood pressure readings of 120–139/80–89 mm Hg (29). This new classification of prehypertension emphasizes the need for more frequent monitoring because prehypertensive individuals are at increased risk for hypertension. The higher the blood pressure, the greater the risk of heart failure (28). In patients with diabetes or renal disease, the blood pressure goal is <120/80 mm Hg (30). Weight reduction results in reduced blood pressure (28); however, some medications for weight loss, high levels of stress, and other factors may increase it.

The mechanism for the relationship between obesity and hypertension is still unclear. Sympathetic activity is increased during overfeeding and decreased during fasting. This sympathetic stimulation is thought to be one reason why hypertension is so prevalent in the obese population. Both visceral fat and insulin resistance seem to be strongly related to hypertension. Sodium retention, which can enhance renal sodium retention and aldosterone secretion, may also be a cause of hypertension in the obese (31). Abnormal vascular responses and alterations in cation transport may be implicated as well. Therefore, weight loss has a significant effect on blood pressure, as well as on insulin resistance. As in most disease states, a 10% weight loss has a significant effect on improvement of hypertension, but more weight loss continues to lower the blood pressure further in those who are responsive.

> *Example:* MA is taking antihypertensive medications. Over the last 6 weeks, he has lost 7% of his body weight (he weighed 225 lb and now weighs 209 lb). He complains about some fatigue and dizziness, but otherwise he is very pleased with his progress and enthusiastic about increasing his exercise routine. The dietetics professional's ears should perk up: MA has new symptoms—dizziness and fatigue. Could they be diet related? Could weight loss have lowered his blood pressure too much? When was the last time his blood pressure was checked?

Team Protocol. In such a case, prompt the client to return to his or her physician's office for an evaluation immediately, and call the physician to confirm. Explain that you are concerned that there has been a change in the blood pressure and you feel uncomfortable about further weight loss until the patient gets reevaluated.

> *Example:* On his first visit, MA did not know his exact blood pressure, but he told you that his physician thought his blood pressure was fine. In the assessment, you took his word at face value and, because he was following ADA guidelines for a safe, moderate 1,500-kcal diet, you felt it was up to his physician and MA to decide whether his blood pressure was within normal limits. However, it is important to consider two issues: (1) some physician offices are not equipped with large enough cuffs to measure blood pressure accurately; and (2) when a patient is borderline and there are no other cardiac risks, the physician may be willing to let the blood pressure go until the next visit. But suppose MA had not seen the physician in 6 months? Suppose he is complaining of occasional headaches?

Team Protocol. In the example above, send MA back to his physician with a note saying that MA has been complaining of headaches. It is helpful to give a description of the dietary regimen, adherence, and weight loss as well. Explain that, because of the patient's complaints of headaches, you are concerned that there may be changes in the blood pressure and that you hope the physician will evaluate the situation and let you know.

Gallbladder Disease

Cholelithiasis is the most common disease associated with overweight, but many patients will present without history of gallbladder disease. Although age, degree of overweight, and female gender increase the risk of gallbladder disease, many people do not have symptoms (32). Furthermore, weight loss, particularly rapid weight loss, and very-low-calorie diets are all promoters of gallbladder disease (33). Although diagnosis can be made by sonogram, it is rarely done because (1) it is difficult to get reimbursement for a "rule-out" diagnosis; and (2) in obese patients, particularly those with abdominal adiposity, a sonogram may be obscured by fat deposits. A physician can prescribe a bile acid, such as ursodeoxycholic acid, as a preventive, but this has not been shown to be effective in weight-loss studies, nor is it indicated as a preventive treatment.

Gallstones in obese people are caused by cholesterol production that is linearly related to body fat. Approximately 20 mg of additional cholesterol is produced for each kilogram of extra body fat. Therefore, there is an increase in cholesterol flow to the bile, causing a supersaturation. But there is no compensatory increase in bile acids or phospholipids, causing a higher risk of cholesterol-type gallstones to precipitate in the gallbladder. During weight loss, there is a greater flux of fats and lipids, causing an increased risk of gallstones. In low-fat diets, there is sometimes a gallbladder stasis that may cause risk as well, particularly when the patient returns to a more liberal food intake (33,34).

> *Example:* SR is a woman you have seen six times in 3 months. She has no history of gallbladder disease. She is 46 years old and has been on "every diet you can imagine" for the last 20 years. Based on sensible guidelines, she has lost 37 pounds in 12 weeks. She is ecstatic, as are you. On the sixth visit, as she is telling you about her food and her social issues, she casually complains about what she thinks is "gas" somewhere, vaguely in the mid-to-upper chest area. She does not dwell on the issue and continues talking about something else. The next time you hear from her, she has to cancel her appointment because she has gallbladder disease. Her primary care physician is sending her to a specialist to decide whether surgery is necessary.

Team Protocol. Symptoms of gallbladder disease can manifest themselves as pain in the upper right or central area of the chest area. If a patient is older than 40 years, with a history of dieting, you should (1) inform the patient that another weight-loss diet increases risk of gallbladder disease; (2) reiterate the risk of rapid weight loss (>1% weight per week) and monitor the rate of weight loss; (3) if using a formula diet or a very-low-fat diet, add 11 grams of fat (2 teaspoons of fat) at one meal per day to stimulate the gall-bladder.

Nonalcoholic Fatty Liver Disease

Nonalcoholic fatty liver disease affects 10% to 25% of the general adult population and 58% to 74% of the obese population (35). What does this mean, and what do nonphysicians have to know? A percentage of these patients go on to steatotic hepatitis (NASH), an irreversible process of fibrosis in the liver.

When a patient, particularly a man, has abdominal obesity, laboratory results often reveal elevated AST and ALT results. Alkaline phosphatase is usually normal without symptoms. Hepatomegaly may be revealed during examination.

> *Example:* HR is a 35-year-old man, with a BMI of 37 and a waist of 103 cm. His cholesterol is 233 mg/dL, which he would like to reduce with diet. His liver function tests are slightly elevated.

Obesity is associated with a significantly greater flow of fatty acids through the portal vein into the liver. There is more lipid stored in the hepatocytes, which causes the liver to become fatty. Likewise, the degree of fatty infiltration usually decreases with weight loss. It is possible to observe short-term increases in AST and ALT as the flux of lipid is increased, but within a short time this is reduced. Rapid weight loss may promote hepatic inflammation.

Team Protocol. If the liver function tests (LFTs) are elevated at the first visit, send the patient back to the physician for evaluation of LFTs within 5 weeks of weight loss, to make sure that the LFTs are reduced.

Final Note

No matter what comorbid conditions exist before treatment, weight loss will likely improve those conditions. However, weight loss comes with some risks. Therefore, it behooves professionals who treat obese patients to work together to build a treatment paradigm (see Box 3B.4).

The strength of the team lies in its ability to learn from each other, acknowledge when to monitor more intensively, and refer to the other members of the team when appropriate. Only then does the team really have a

Box 3B.4. The Patient's Team

Nonphysician Responsibilities

Monitor: Rate of weight loss, changes in clinical status, physical complaints, compliance, visits to the physician.

Reevaluate: The effect of the diet, the patient's nutrition intake, success lifestyle changes, plateaus.

Behavior: Ask about successes and other needs of support; encourage access to the nonphysician as needed.

Physician Responsibilities

Monitor: Blood pressure, heart rate, lab work, any physical complaints.

Reevaluate: Medications, health profile, frequency of visits, weight loss, the team's success, any changes in dietary regimen.

Behavior: Ask about successes and other needs of support; encourage access to the physician as needed.

protocol, a measurable direction in which there is a better opportunity to avoid the pitfalls. And only then can the team provide the best care.

References

1. Sciamanna CN, Tate DF, Lang W, Wing RR. Who reports receiving advice to lose weight? Results from a multistate survey. *Arch Intern Med.* 2000;160:2334–2339.
2. Centers for Obesity Research and Education. Weighing the Risks (unpublished handout). Denver, Colo: Centers for Obesity Research and Education.
3. Cummings S, Parham ES, Strain GW. Position of the American Dietetic Association: weight management. *J Am Diet Assoc.* 2002;108:1146–1155.
4. El-Kebbi IM, Cook CB, Ziemer DC, Miller CD, Gallina DL, Phillips LS. Association of younger age with poor glycemic control and obesity in urban African Americans with type 2 diabetes. *Arch Intern Med.* 2003;163:69–75.
5. National Institutes of Health: National Heart, Lung and Blood Institute: North American Association for the Study of Obesity. *The Practical Guide: Identification, Evaluation and Treatment of Overweight and Obesity in Adults.* Rockville, Md: National Institutes of Health; 2000. NIH Publication No. 00-4084.
6. Elia M. Obesity in the elderly. *Obes Res.* 2001;9(Suppl 4):S244–S248.
7. Ryan AS, Nicklas BJ, Berman DM. Racial differences in insulin resistance and mid-thigh fat deposition in postmenopausal women. *Obes Res.* 2002;10:336–344.

8. Garrow JS. Composition of weight loss during therapeutic dietary restriction. In: Kral JG, Van Itallie TB, eds. *Recent Developments in Body Composition Analysis: Methods and Applications*. London, England: Smith-Gordon; 1993: 121–127.

9. Van Itallie TB, Yang MU. Diet and weight loss. *N Engl J Med*. 1977;297: 1158–1161.

10. Yang MU, Van Itallie TB. Effect of energy restriction on body composition and nitrogen balance in obese individuals. In: Wadden TA, Van Itallie TB, eds. *Treatment of the Seriously Obese Patient*. New York, NY: Guilford Press; 1992:83–106.

11. Nonas CA. A model for chronic care of obesity through dietary treatment. *J Am Diet Assoc*. 1998; 98(Suppl 2):S16–S22.

12. Rathmann W, Funkhouser E, Dyer AR, Roseman JM. Relations of hyperuricemia with the various components of the insulin resistance syndrome in young black and white adults: the CARDIA study. Coronary Artery Risk Development in Young Adults. *Ann Epidemiol*. 1998;4:250–261.

13. St. Jeor ST, Howard BV, Prewitt TE, Bovee V, Bazzarre T, Eckel RH. Dietary protein and weight reduction: a statement for healthcare professionals from the Nutrition Committee of the Council on Nutrition, Physical Activity, and Metabolism of the American Heart Association. *Circulation*. 2001;104: 1869–1874.

14. Pi-Sunyer FX. Short-term medical benefits and adverse effects of weight loss. *Ann Intern Med*. 1993;119:722–726.

15. Nonas C, PiSunyer FX, Foster GD. Obese women with metabolic syndrome. In: *Medical Nutrition and Disease*. 3rd ed. Malden, Mass: Blackwell Publishing; 2003:25–38.

16. Knowler WC, Barrett-Connor E, Fowler SE, Hamman RF, Lachin JM, Walker EA, Nathan DM. Reduction in the incidence of type 2 diabetes with lifestyle intervention or metformin. *New Engl J Med*. 2002;346:393–403.

17. Flemons WF. Obstructive sleep apnea. *N Engl J Med*. 2002;347:498–504.

18. Young T, Palta M, Dempsey J, Skatrud J, Weber S, Badr S. The occurrence of sleep-disordered breathing among middle-aged adults. *N Engl J Med*. 1993;328:1230–1235.

19. Strobel RJ, Rosen RC. Obesity and weight loss in obstructive sleep apnea: a critical review. *Sleep*. 1996;19:104–115.

20. Kenchaiah S, Evans JC, Levy D, Wilson PW, Benjamin EJ, Larson MG, Kannel WB, Vasan RS. Obesity and the risk of heart failure. *N Engl J Med*. 2002;347: 305–359.

21. Redfield MM. Heart failure—an epidemic of uncertain proportions. *N Engl J Med*. 2002;347:1442–1444.

22. Saltzman E, Benotti PN. The effects of obesity on the cardiovascular system. In: Bray GA, Bouchard C, James WPT, eds. *Handbook of Obesity*. New York, NY: Marcel Dekker; 1998:637–649.

23. Albert MA, Lambert CR, Terry BE, Cohen MV, Mukerji V, Massey CV, Hashimi MW, Panayiotou H. Interrelationship of left ventricular mass, systolic function, and diastolic filling in normotensive morbidly obese patients. *Int J Obes Relat Metab Disord*.1995;19:550–557.

24. Pietrobelli A, Rothacker D, Gallagher D, Heymsfield SB. Electrocardiographic QTC interval: short-term weight loss effects. *Int J Obes Relat Metab Disord.* 1997;21:110–114.

25. Fisler JS. Cardiac effects of starvation and semistarvation diets: safety and mechanism of action. *Am J Clin Nutr.* 1992;56(Suppl 1):230S–234S.

26. Third Report of the National Cholesterol Education Program (NCEP) Expert Panel on Detection, Evaluation, and Treatment of High Blood Cholesterol in Adults (Adult Treatment Panel III) final report. *Circulation.* 2002;106:3143–3421.

27. Chobanian AV, Bakris GL, Black HR, Cushman WC, Green LA, Izzo JL Jr, Jones DW, Materson BJ, Oparil S, Wright JT Jr, Roccella EJ; National Heart, Lung, and Blood Institute Joint National Committee on Prevention, Detection, Evaluation, and Treatment of High Blood Pressure; National High Blood Pressure Education Program Coordinating Committee. The Seventh Report of the Joint National Committee on Prevention, Detection, Evaluation, and Treatment of High Blood Pressure: the JNC 7 report. *JAMA* 2003;289:2573–2575.

28. Brown CD, Higgins M, Donato KA, Rohde FC, Garrison R, Obarzanek E, Ernst ND, Horan M. Body mass index and the prevalence of hypertension and dyslipidemia. *Obes Res.* 2000;9:605–619.

29. Whelton PK, He J, Appel LJ, Cutler JA, Havas S, Kotchen TA, Roccella EJ, Stout R, Vallbona C, Winston MC, Karimbakas J; National High Blood Pressure Education Program Coordinating Committee. Primary prevention of hypertension: clinical and public health advisory from The National High Blood Pressure Education Program. *JAMA.*2002;288:1882–1888.

30. Chobanian AV, Bakris GL, Black HR, Cushman WC, Green LA, Izzo JL, Jones DW, Materson BJ, Oparil S, Wright JT, Roccella EJ; the National High Blood Pressure Education Program Coordinating Committee. The Seventh Report of the Joint National Committee on Prevention, Detection, Evaluation, and Treatment of High Blood Pressure. *JAMA.* 2003;289:2560–2571.

31. Rocchini AP. Obesity and blood pressure regulation. In: Bray GA, Bouchard C, James WPT, eds. *Handbook of Obesity.* New York, NY: Marcel Dekker; 1998:677–696.

32. Stampfer MJ, Maclure KM, Colditz GA, Manson JE, Willett WC. Risk of symptomatic gallstones in women with severe obesity. *Am J Clin Nutr.* 1992; 55:652–658.

33. Liddle RA, Goldstein RB, Saxton J. Gallstone formation during weight-reduction dieting. *Arch Int Med.* 1989;149:1750–1753.

34. Ko CW, Lee SP. Obesity and gallbladder disease. In: Bray GA, Bouchard C, James WP, eds. *Handbook of Obesity.* New York, NY: Marcel Dekker; 1998: 677–695.

35. Angulo P. Nonalcoholic fatty liver disease. *N Engl J Med.* 2002;346:1221–1231.

Chapter 4

Behavioral Treatment

PART A. Overview

Thomas A. Wadden, PhD

An expert panel convened by the National Heart, Lung, and Blood Institute (NHLBI) recently completed an exhaustive review of treatments for obesity (1). The panel recommended that obese individuals initially attempt to lose weight through a combination of low-calorie diet, regular physical activity, and behavior therapy. Although the first two interventions are well known to the public and health professionals, behavior therapy is not. It refers to a set of principles and techniques for adopting new eating, activity, and thinking habits (2). This chapter briefly describes behavior therapy's defining characteristics, its treatment results, and its application in clinical practice. The terms "behavior therapy" and "behavior modification" are used interchangeably in this chapter, as they are by most professionals. Two additional terms—"behavioral treatment" and "lifestyle modification"—are frequently used to describe the combination of approaches (including diet, exercise, and behavior therapy) used to induce weight loss.

Behavior Therapy for Obesity: Overview

Historically, behavioral treatment developed from the belief that obesity was the result of maladaptive eating and exercise habits (3). These habits were thought to be learned and could be corrected by the application of learning principles. Today, investigators realize that body weight is affected by factors other than behavior. These include genetic, metabolic, and hormonal influences (4–7) that probably predispose some persons to obesity and may well set the range of possible weights that an individual can achieve. Some individuals may never be thin, despite their most heroic efforts to modify eating and activity habits. Behavior therapy, however, can help such individuals develop a set of skills (such as eating a low-calorie, low-fat diet) to achieve a healthier weight, even if they cannot attain an ideal one.

Behavioral treatment is based largely on principles of classical conditioning, which posit that eating is often prompted by antecedent events (ie, cues) that become strongly linked to food intake (3). For example, the sight and smell of food alone often arouse appetite, because of their repeated pairing with the pleasurable sensations (eg, taste and fullness) of eating. Food advertisements capitalize on this conditioning. Similarly, eating may become paired with cues that include negative emotions, watching television, or socializing with friends (8,9). The more often two events are paired together, the stronger the connection between them, so that the presence of one automatically triggers the other. This explains the frequent desire for popcorn when entering a movie theater. Behavioral treatment, as described below, helps patients identify cues that trigger inappropriate eating (and activity) and learn new responses to them (8,9).

Treatment also seeks to reinforce (or reward) the adoption of positive behaviors, while also reducing the aversiveness associated with some types of behavior change. In the first case, parents might praise their overweight son every time he ate more fruits and vegetables and could provide him with a small gift at the end of the week (10). With time, the son might find that he enjoyed the taste of apples and bananas, making these foods rewarding in themselves. In the second case, a patient might state that she disliked exercising because of physical exhaustion or pain, consequences that are likely to derail any exercise plan. She would be encouraged to find an activity that she enjoyed (such as walking) and initially undertake it at a low intensity for brief periods (11). Her activity would be increased gradually, to ensure that it did not cause discomfort.

In the last 20 years, cognitive therapy has also been incorporated in the behavioral treatment of obesity. The underlying assumption of cognitive therapy is that thoughts (or cognitions) directly affect feelings and behaviors (12). Negative thoughts frequently are associated with negative outcomes, as in the case of a man who overeats, tells himself he's "blown his diet," and then proceeds to eat triple the original amount because of feelings of disgust and despair. With cognitive therapy, patients learn to set realistic goals for weight and behavior change, to evaluate their success in modifying eating and activity habits, and to correct negative thoughts that occur when they do not meet their goals (9,13,14). Cognitive interventions for weight management are based on those developed for the treatments of depression, anxiety, and bulimia nervosa (15–17).

Defining Characteristics

Behavioral treatment has several distinguishing characteristics (2). First, it is goal directed. It specifies very clear goals in terms that can be easily measured. This is true whether the goal is walking four times a week, lengthening meal duration by 10 minutes, or decreasing the number of self-critical comments. Specific goals facilitate a clear assessment of success.

Second, treatment is process oriented. It is more than helping people to decide what to change (eg, eating, activity, or thinking habits); it is helping them to identify how to change (2). Thus, once a goal is specified, patients are encouraged to examine factors that will facilitate or hinder goal achievement. In cases in which the desired behavior is not implemented, problem-solving skills are used to identify new strategies to overcome barriers. In this view, successful weight management is based on skills that can be learned and practiced, in the same manner that an individual can learn to play the piano through frequent practice. Skill power, not will power, is the key to success.

Third, the behavioral approach advocates small rather than large changes. This is based on the learning principle of successive approximation, in which incremental steps are taken to achieve more distant goals. Making small changes gives patients successful experiences upon which to build rather than attempting drastic changes that are typically short-lived.

The Behavioral Package

Behavioral treatment usually includes multiple components, such as keeping food and activity records (ie, self-monitoring), controlling cues associated with eating (ie, stimulus control), nutrition education, slowing eating, physical activity, problem solving, and cognitive restructuring (ie, cognitive therapy) (8,9). These components comprise the "behavioral package," which has been summarized in manuals such as the *LEARN Program for Weight Management 2000* (9). Studies have shown that two components—self-monitoring (18,19) and physical activity (20,21)—are consistently associated with better weight control, short- and long-term, respectively. Surprisingly, there is little empirical evidence to support the use of stimulus control, problem solving, or cognitive restructuring, either because the necessary studies have not been conducted or negative results were obtained. Further research clearly is needed to identify the most potent components of the package, as well as additional interventions that might be added (such as body-image therapy) (22). In the interim, researchers and practitioners probably will continue to use the behavioral package, because it is well validated, as a whole, and different patients are drawn to different components of the intervention.

Structure of Treatment

The structure of behavioral treatment may be as important as its contents. Participants typically attend weekly group meetings of 60 to 90 minutes that are led by a registered dietitian, a behavioral psychologist, an exercise physiologist, or some other health professional. Group sessions appear to provide a combination of social support and friendly competition (2). The weekly weigh-in is a major motivator for participants, who compare their weight losses (either formally or informally) with those of other group members. A recent study found that group treatment induced larger initial weight losses than individual treatment (23). This was true even for patients who indicated that they preferred individual treatment but were randomly assigned to receive group care. They lost more weight than persons who preferred individual treatment and received it.

Results of Behavioral Treatment

Short-term Results

Reviews of the literature have consistently shown that patients treated by a comprehensive-group behavioral approach lose approximately 8.5 kg (about 9% of initial weight) in 20 to 26 weeks of treatment (2,8,24). Approximately 80% of patients who begin treatment complete it. Thus, behavioral treatment yields very favorable results, as judged by criteria proposed by the NHLBI expert panel (1), as well as by the World Health Organization (WHO) (25) and the Institute of Medicine of the National Academy of Sciences (26). Most behaviorally treated participants will lose at least 5% to 10% of initial weight, a loss associated with reductions in cardiovascular risk factors.

The mean loss of 9% of initial weight, described above, was achieved with the prescription of a 1,200- to 1,500-kcal/day diet of conventional foods. Obese individuals typically underestimate their calorie intake by 20% to 40% when consuming a diet of conventional foods (27,28). Recent studies have shown that weight losses increase significantly with the prescription of portion-controlled meals that provide dieters a premeasured amount of food with a known energy content (29). Liquid meal replacements, such as SlimFast (30,31), are examples of such an approach, as are frozen food entrees. Portion-controlled meals facilitate adherence to calorie goals. Wadden et al (32), for example, found that participants who consumed a 950-kcal/day diet, comprised of liquid meal replacements and frozen food entrees, lost an average of 14.4 kg in 4 months. Weight losses also are increased by giving participants portion-controlled servings of conventional foods or simply by providing detailed menus of foods to be consumed (29,33).

Long-term Results

Participants treated by a comprehensive behavioral approach regain approximately one third of their lost weight in the year after treatment, with increasing regain over time. At 5 years after treatment, participants, on average, return to their baseline weight. Although disappointing, such results are not entirely unexpected. Twenty weekly group sessions are no match, in the long-term, for Americans' sedentary lifestyle or for the food industry's multibillion-dollar-per-year advertising budget (34,35). This toxic environment, as Brownell has named it (35), contributes not only to weight regain but to the epidemic of obesity itself.

Several interventions improve the maintenance of weight loss (see Chapter 9: Weight-Loss Maintenance). The first is to recognize that obesity is a chronic disorder that requires long-term care, one form of which is continued patient-provider contact after initial weight loss (36). Perri et al, for example, found that patients who attended group maintenance sessions every other week for the year after treatment maintained 13.0 kg of their 13.2-kg weight loss (37). Patients who did not receive such therapy maintained only 5.7 kg of a 10.8-kg loss. Patient-provider contact may also be provided by telephone or mail (38). Maintenance of weight loss is also facilitated by the long-term use of medications, including sibutramine (39) and orlistat (40) (see Chapter 7: Pharmacological Treatment). A recent study found that orlistat was associated with a 6.4% reduction in initial weight at a 4-year assessment, the longest trial of medication to date.

Long-term Health Consequences of Weight Loss

Multiple investigations have shown that weight losses of 5% to 10% of initial weight, as produced by behavioral treatment, are associated with short-term improvements in hypertension, type 2 diabetes, hypercholesterolemia, and other weight-related complications (1,25,26,41). Results of the Diabetes Prevention Program (DPP) recently provided definitive evidence of the long-term benefits of modest weight loss (42). More than 3,200 overweight (and obese) individuals with impaired glucose tolerance were randomly assigned to (1) placebo, (2) metformin (850 mg bid), or (3) a lifestyle intervention designed to induce a loss of 7% of initial weight and to increase physical activity to at least 150 minutes a week. As shown in Figure 4A.1,

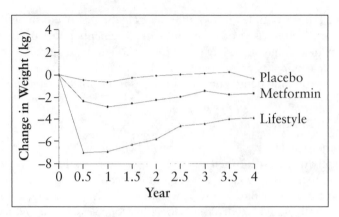

Figure 4A.1. Changes in Body Weight in the Diabetes Prevention Program
    Each data point represents the mean value for all participants examined at that time. The number of participants decreased over time because of the variable length of time that persons were in the study. For example, data on weight were available for 3085 persons at 0.5 year, 3,064 at 1 year, 2,887 at 2 years, and 1,510 at 3 years. Changes in weight over time differed significantly among the treatment groups (P < 0.001 for each comparison).
    Reprinted by permission from Knowler WC, Barrett-Conner E, Fowler SE, Hamman RF, Lachin JM, Walker EA, Nathan DM. Reduction in the incidence of type 2 diabetes with lifestyle intervention or metformin. *New Engl J Med.* 2002;346:393–403. Copyright © 2002 Massachusetts Medical Society. All rights reserved.

lifestyle participants lost an average of 7 kg (approximately 7%) by the end of the first year, compared with essentially no change in the placebo group and a loss of 2 kg in metformin-treated participants. Lifestyle-treated participants also engaged in significantly more physical activity than patients in the two other conditions. These improvements in weight and physical activity were associated with a highly significant reduction in the risk of developing type 2 diabetes (see Figure 4A.2). At the 4-year assessment, lifestyle participants experienced a 58% reduction in risk compared with placebo-treated individuals, and a 38% reduction compared with patients in the metformin group. A recent Finnish study similarly showed that a 5% loss of initial weight significantly reduced the risk of developing type 2 diabetes during a 3- to 4-year period (43).

    Examination of Figures 4A.1 and 4A.2 reveals that even though lifestyle-treated participants regained weight from years 2 to 4, their reduced risk of developing type 2 diabetes was as great at year 4 as at any other time. This finding suggests that overweight and obese individuals should not be deterred from dieting because of concerns that they may regain weight. Weight loss, even if followed by weight regain, appears to be associated with significant health improvements, if the weight loss was intentional (42,44).

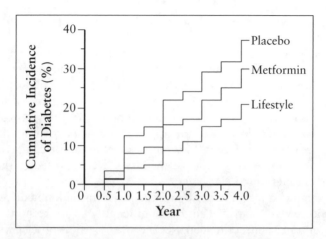

Figure 4A.2. Cumulative Incidence of Diabetes for Participants in the Diabetes Prevention Program

Patients were randomly assigned to placebo, metformin (850 mg/d b.i.d.) or lifestyle modification. The diagnosis of diabetes was based on the criteria of the American Diabetes Association. The incidence of diabetes differed significantly among the 3 groups (*P* < 0.001 for each comparison).

Reprinted by permission from Knowler WC, Barrett-Conner E, Fowler SE, Hamman RF, Lachin JM, Walker EA, Nathan DM. Reduction in the incidence of type 2 diabetes with lifestyle intervention or metformin. *New Engl J Med.* 2002;346:393–403. Copyright © 2002 Massachusetts Medical Society. All rights reserved.

Additional studies have refuted concerns that a cycle of weight loss and regain is associated with adverse effects on resting energy expenditure, body composition, or psychological status (45–47). Similarly, dieting (ie, energy restriction), in overweight individuals, is not associated with the precipitation of binge eating or mood disorders (45,48).

Behavioral Treatment: The Next Generation of Research

The behavioral treatment of obesity, as provided in academic medical centers, clearly is efficacious and is associated with marked improvements in weight-related health complications. Little, however, is known about the effectiveness of behavioral treatment as it might be implemented in primary care practice or in community settings. Unfortunately, such treatment is not available to the millions of Americans who need to lose weight. Fewer than 500 programs nationwide probably offer group treatment, as described previously, and therapy can cost $25 or more per week (and up to $125 per week in medically supervised programs). Thus, investigators must find effective methods of providing behavioral treatment, at an affordable cost, to large numbers of persons.

Promising venues for intervention include worksites, schools, and places of worship (49). Research is needed to determine the personal characteristics and training that group leaders require, in these settings, to deliver effective behavioral treatment (50). Studies have suggested that laypersons may be as effective as professionals in facilitating weight loss, which could significantly reduce the cost of therapy (51). Participants in a self-help behavioral program that received no professional guidance achieved some of the most impressive long-term weight losses ever reported in the weight-management literature (52).

Given the fast pace of modern life, Americans undoubtedly would like "drive-thru weight management," free of lengthy group sessions or significant travel time. This desire increases the attractiveness of telephone- or Internet-based interventions. A recent study by Tate et al reported a loss of 4 kg in 6 months in participants who received an Internet-based behavioral program (53). This is only the beginning of research on off-site interventions. Supermarket self-help, in the form of liquid meal replacements or portion-controlled frozen-food entrees, may also be of benefit, although further studies are needed on this topic (54).

Treatment alone will not be sufficient to reverse our nation's epidemic of obesity. Effectiveness research must be complemented by the application of behavioral principles to the prevention of overweight and obesity (55). This will require health care professionals to address obesity (and decreased physical activity) as a public policy issue in a manner similar to cigarette smoking. Ultimately, we must re-engineer the food and activity environment in our homes, schools, and workplaces, so that they yield healthy children and adults.

References

1. Clinical guidelines on the identification, evaluation, and treatment of overweight and obesity in adults—the evidence report. National Institutes of Health. *Obes Res.* 1998;6:51S–210S.
2. Wadden TA, Foster GD. Behavioral treatment of obesity. *Med Clin North Am.* 2000;84:441–461.
3. Stuart RB. Behavioral control of overeating. *Behav Ther.* 1967;5:357–365.
4. Stunkard AJ, Harris JR, Pedersen NL, McClearn GE. The body-mass index of twins who have been reared apart. *N Engl J Med.* 1990;322:1483–1487.
5. Ravussin E, Lillioja S, Knowler WC, Christin L, Freymond D, Abbott WG, Boyce V, Howard BV, Bogardus C. Reduced rate of energy expenditure as a risk factor for body-weight gain. *N Engl J Med.* 1988;318:467–472.

6. Campfield LA, Smith FJ, Guisez Y, Devos R, Burn P. Recombinant mouse OB protein: evidence for a peripheral signal linking adiposity and central neural networks. *Science*. 1995;269:546–549.
7. Perusse L, Chagnon YC, Dionne FT, Bouchard C. The human obesity gene map: the 1996 update. *Obes Res*. 1997;5:49–61.
8. Wing RR. Behavioral weight control. In: Wadden TA, Stunkard AJ, eds. *Handbook of Obesity Treatment*. New York, NY: Guilford; 2002:301–316.
9. Brownell KD. *The LEARN Program for Weight Management 2000: Lifestyle, Exercise, Attitudes, Relationships, Nutrition*. Dallas, Tex: American Health Publishing Co; 2000.
10. Epstein LH. Family-based behavioural intervention for obese children. *Int J Obes Relat Metab Disord*. 1996;20:S14–S21.
11. Andersen RE, Wadden TA, Bartlett SJ, Zemel B, Verde TJ, Franckowiak SC. Effects of lifestyle activity vs. structured aerobic exercise in obese women: a randomized trial. *JAMA*. 1999;281:335–340.
12. Beck AT. *Cognitive Therapy and the Emotional Disorder*. New York, NY: International Universities Press; 1976.
13. Foster GD. Goals and strategies to improve behavior-change effectiveness. In: Bessesen DH, Kushner RF, eds. *Evaluation and Management of Obesity*. Philadelphia, Pa: Hanley & Belfus; 2002:29–32.
14. Foster GD, Wadden TA, Vogt RA, Brewer G. What is a reasonable weight loss? Patients' expectations and evaluations of obesity treatment outcomes. *J Consult Clin Psychol*. 1997;65:79–85.
15. Beck AT. *Cognitive Therapy of Depression*. New York, NY: Guilford Press; 1979.
16. Beck AT, Emery G, Greenberg RL. *Anxiety Disorders and Phobias: A Cognitive Perspective*. New York, NY: Basic Books; 1985.
17. Fairburn CG, Wilson GT. *Binge Eating: Nature, Assessment, and Treatment*. New York, NY: Guilford Press; 1993.
18. Baker RC, Kirschenbaum DS. Self-monitoring may be necessary for successful weight control. *Behav Ther*. 1993;24:377–394.
19. Jeffery RW, Bjornson-Benson WM, Rosenthal BS, Lindquist RA, Kurth CL, Johnson SL. Correlates of weight loss and its maintenance over two years of follow-up among middle-aged men. *Prev Med*. 1984;13:155–168.
20. Kayman S, Bruvold W, Stern JS. Maintenance and relapse after weight loss in women: behavioral aspects. *Am J Clin Nutr*. 1990;52:800–807.
21. Wing RR, Hill JO. Successful weight loss maintenance. *Annu Rev Nutr*. 2001; 21:323–341.
22. Rosen JC, Orosan P, Reiter J. Cognitive behavior therapy for negative body image in obese women. *Behav Ther*. 1995;26:25–42.
23. Renjilian DA, Perri MG, Nezu AM, Mckelvey WF, Shermer RL, Anton SD. Individual versus group therapy for obesity: effects of matching participants to their treatment preferences. *J Consult Clin Psychol*. 2001;69:717–721.
24. Wadden TA. Treatment of obesity by moderate and severe caloric restriction. Results of clinical research trials. *Ann Intern Med*. 1993;119:688–693.
25. World Health Organization. *Obesity: Preventing and Managing the Global Epidemic: Report of a WHO Consultation*. Geneva, Switzerland; 2000.

26. Thomas PR. *Weighing the Options: Criteria for Evaluating Weight-Management Programs*. Washington, DC: National Academy Press; 1995.
27. Lichtman SW, Pisarka K, Berman ER, Pestone M, Dowling H, Offenbacher E, Weisel H, Heshka S, Matthews DE, Heymsfield SB. Discrepancy between self-reported and actual caloric intake and exercise in obese subjects. *N Engl J Med*. 1992;327:1893–1898.
28. Bandini LG, Schoeller DA, Cyr HN, Dietz WH. Validity of reported energy intake in obese and nonobese adolescents. *Am J Clin Nutr*. 1990;52:421–425.
29. Jeffery RW, Wing RR, Thornson C, Burton LR, Raether C, Harvey J, Mullen M. Strengthening behavioral interventions for weight loss: a randomized trial of food provision and monetary incentives. *J Consult Clin Psychol*. 1993;61:1038–1045.
30. Ditschuneit HH, Flechtner-Mors M, Johnson TD, Adler G. Metabolic and weight-loss effects of long-term dietary intervention in obese subjects. *Am J Clin Nutr*. 1999;69:198–204.
31. Ashley JM, St. Jeor ST, Schrage JP, Perumean-Chaney SE, Gilbertson MC, McCall NL, Bovee V. Weight control in the physician's office. *Arch Intern Med*. 2001;161:1599–1604.
32. Wadden TA, Vogt RA, Andersen RE, Bartlett SJ, Foster GD, Kuehnel RH, Wilk J, Weinstock R, Buckenmeyer P, Berkowitz RI, Steen SN. Exercise in the treatment of obesity: effects of four interventions on body composition, resting energy expenditure, appetite and mood. *J Consult Clin Psychol*. 1997;65:269–277.
33. Wing RR, Jeffery RW, Burton LR, Thorson C, Nissinoff K, Baxter JE. Food provisions vs structured meal plans in the behavioral treatment of obesity. *Int J Obes Relat Metab Disord*. 1996;20:56–62.
34. Hill JO, Peters JC. Environmental contributions to the obesity epidemic. *Science*. 1998;280:1371–1374.
35. Horgen KB, Brownell KD. Confronting the toxic environment: environmental, public health actions in a world crisis. In: Wadden TA, Stunkard AJ, eds. *Handbook of Obesity Treatment*. New York, NY: Guilford Press; 2002:95–106.
36. Perri MG, Sears SF, Clark JE. Strategies for improving maintenance of weight loss: toward a continuous care model of obesity management. *Diabetes Care*. 1993;16:200–209.
37. Perri MG, McAllister DA, Gange JJ, Jordan RC, McAdoo WG, Nezu AM. Effects of four maintenance programs on the long-term management of obesity. *J Consult Clin Psychol*. 1988;56:529–534.
38. Perri MG, Shapiro RM, Ludwig WW, Twentyman CT, McAdoo WG. Maintenance strategies for the treatment of obesity: an evaluation of relapse prevention training and posttreatment contact by mail and telephone. *J Consult Clin Psychol*. 1984;52:404–413.
39. James WP, Astrup A, Finer N, Hilsted J, Kopelman P, Rossner S, Saris WH, Van Gaal LF. Effect of sibutramine on weight maintenance after weight loss: a randomised trial. STORM Study Group. Sibutramine Trial of Obesity Reduction and Maintenance. *Lancet*. 2000;356:2119–2125.

40. Sjostrom L, Rissanen A, Andersen T, Boldrin M, Golay A, Koppeschaar HP, Krempf M. Randomised placebo-controlled trial of orlistat for weight loss and prevention of weight regain in obese patients. *Lancet.* 1998;352:167–172.
41. Goldstein DJ. Beneficial health effects of moderate weight loss. *Int J Obes Relat Metab Disord.* 1992;16:397–415.
42. Knowler WC, Barrett-Conner E, Fowler SE, Hamman RF, Lachin JM, Walker EA, Nathan DM. Reduction in the incidence of type 2 diabetes with lifestyle intervention or metformin. *New Engl J Med.* 2002;346:393–403.
43. Tuomilehto J, Lindstrom J, Eriksson JG, Valle TT, Hamalainen H, Ilanne-Parikka P, Keinanen-Kiukaanniemi S, Laakso M, Louheranta A, Rastas M, Salminen V, Uusitupa M. Prevention of type 2 diabetes mellitus by changes in lifestyle among subjects with impaired glucose tolerance. *New Engl J Med.* 2001;344:1343–1350.
44. Wing RR, Jeffery RW, Hellerstedt WL. A prospective study of effects of weight cycling on cardiovascular risk factors. *Arch Intern Med.* 1995;155:1416–1422.
45. Foster GD, Wadden TA, Kendall PC, Stunkard AJ, Vogt RA. Psychological effects of weight loss and regain: a prospective evaluation. *J Consult Clin Psychol.* 1996;64:752–757.
46. Wadden TA, Foster GD, Stunkard AJ, Conill AM. Effects of weight cycling on the resting energy expenditure and body composition of obese women. *Int J Eat Disord.* 1996;19:5–12.
47. National Task Force on the Prevention and Treatment of Obesity. Weight cycling. *JAMA.* 1994;272:1196–1202.
48. Dieting and the development of eating disorders in overweight and obese adults. *Arch Intern Med.* 2000;160:2581–2589.
49. Schmitz KH, Jeffery JW. Prevention of obesity. In: Wadden TA, Stunkard AJ, eds. *Handbook of Obesity Treatment.* New York, NY: Guilford Press; 2002:556–593.
50. Wang SS, Wadden TA, Womble LG, Nonas CA. What consumers want to know about commercial weight-loss programs: a pilot investigation. *Obes Res.* 2003;11:48–53.
51. Brownell KD, Stunkard AJ, McKeon PE. Weight reduction at the worksite: a promise partially fulfilled. *Am J Psychiatry.* 1985;142:47–52.
52. Latner JD, Stunkard AJ, Wilson GT, Jackson ML, Zelitch DS, Labouvie E. Effective long-term treatment of obesity: a continuing care model. *Int J Obes.* 2000;24:893–898.
53. Tate DF, Wing RR, Winett RA. Using Internet technology to deliver a behavioral weight loss program. *JAMA.* 2001;285;1172–1177.
54. Womble LG, Wang SS, Wadden TA. Commercial and self-help weight loss programs. In: Wadden TA, Stunkard AJ, eds. *Handbook of Obesity Treatment.* New York, NY: Guilford Press, 2002:395–415.
55. Wadden TA, Brownell KD, Foster GD. Obesity: responding to the global epidemic. *J Consult Clin Psychol.* 2002;70:510–525.

PART B. Practical Applications

Gary D. Foster, PhD, and Angie Makris, PhD, RD

The behavioral treatment of obesity consists of methods to help patients make long-term changes in eating, activity, and thought patterns (see Part A of this chapter). It is the cornerstone of any dietary, pharmacological, or surgical treatment of obesity. This chapter reviews practical aspects of implementing behavioral strategies in the clinical setting.

Setting the Stage

Talking With Patients About Weight Control

No matter what type of obesity treatment is ultimately recommended, effective and compassionate treatment of obese patients requires an understanding of the cultural context in which treatment occurs. As Stunkard and Sobal have suggested, disparagement of obese individuals is the last socially acceptable form of prejudice (1). It is not surprising, therefore, that health care providers seem to share society's negative view of the overweight. Studies suggest that a large proportion of physicians consider obesity a behavioral problem (ie, resulting from lack of willpower or lack of physical activity) and view obese patients as lazy, awkward, unattractive, and ugly (2,3). Other health care providers, including registered dietitians, also have negative or at best ambivalent attitudes toward obese persons (4–7). Such characterizations are likely to lead to behaviors that may be discriminatory. There are numerous clinical anecdotes about how obese patients have been treated disrespectfully in the health care setting.

Toward More Empathic Encounters.   It can be argued that overweight patients are "just too sensitive," and their perceptions about medical visits reflect their own frustration with their weight rather than any systemic bias by health care professionals. Even if patients' bad experiences are partly a result of their inaccurate perceptions, such experiences need to be remedied. This is necessary because these inaccurate perceptions lead to interactions that, at best, provide health care at the expense of a patient's self-esteem or, at worst, prevent obese patients from seeking health care altogether. The following recommendations seek to put obese patients at ease in the health care setting and to promote competent, compassionate care (8):

- *Assume that obese individuals know they are overweight.* If they have not heard it from a health care professional, they have probably been told by friends, family, or even strangers. Simple phrases such as, "What do you think about your weight?" will allow you to assess the patient's interest and/or motivation for weight control in a *nonjudgmental* fashion. They also allow you to hear the patient's perspective before making any recommendations for weight loss or describing the ill effects of excess weight.
- *Be empathic about dissatisfaction with weight and/or shape.* It is reassuring for patients to hear from their health care providers things like, "Weight control is really tough work, isn't it?" or, "It must be frustrating to have worked so hard and still be unhappy because you haven't lost as much weight as you wanted." Such phrases let patients know that you understand their difficulties and that you will not be judgmental.
- *Listen carefully to the patient's presenting problem, independent of weight.* Few patients consider weight to be their primary problem. As Stunkard points out, patients define the presenting problem (9). If weight is a precipitating condition, focus on the factors that affect the presenting problem *and* weight. For example, it is not useful to tell an obese patient with dyslipidemia to lose weight. Encouraging the same patient to decrease the intake of saturated fat and make small changes in activity, however, will likely influence weight and lipids.

Creating a Receptive Environment

Just as airline seats are frequently too small for significantly obese patients, so are the equipment and furnishings found in many health care settings. Attention to the following details facilitates an environment that is receptive to obese patients:

- *Have a scale that can weigh all patients.* Getting weighed is among the most unpleasant experiences for an obese patient in the health care setting; it becomes humiliating if a patient weighs more than the scale can accommodate.
- *Have gowns available that fit larger patients.* Many obese patients report the experience of waiting for a physician examination in a gown that barely covers them.
- *Use larger blood pressure cuffs when appropriate.* Office and/or hospital staff should know when to use larger cuffs with patients. Inappropriate cuff sizes will lead to inaccurate measurements and treatment recommendations. Moreover, having a cuff inflate off a patient's arm is awkward for both the patient and the practitioner.
- *Provide some armless chairs in the waiting room.* Obese patients should not be made to feel uncomfortable in chairs made for lean persons.

Counseling Skills

Although behavioral change is the responsibility of the patient, the health care provider can facilitate change through effective counseling. Counseling involves both nonverbal skills (eg, eye contact, body language, tone of voice) and verbal ones (10). Counseling is not an innate talent; it requires practice and fine-tuning.

Open vs Closed Questions

Many times during counseling sessions, health care providers fall into the trap of asking closed questions (eg, eliciting a "yes," "no," or single-word response) or questions beginning with "why." Unless the goal is to obtain straightforward information (eg, medical history), these types of questions should be avoided. Asking "why" can be useful at times, but it may also put a patient on the defensive or result in a "dead-end" response (eg, "I don't know") (10). Open-ended questions (eg, "*What* changes do you think you'll have to make in order to lose weight?" or "*How* do you think each family member could be more supportive?" or "*Tell me more* about wanting to make a fresh start.") and reflective statements (eg, "*It sounds like* you've been frustrated with your weight for a long time.") generate more information from the patient than closed questions. Such information encourages collaboration and helps clinicians better understand a patient's point of view.

Content vs Process

Suppose a patient comes to the office after several weeks of dietary and behavioral counseling and has not lost weight. What would your first instinct lead you to do? Would you first review the patient's food record, evaluate food selection, assess accuracy of record keeping, or inquire about the patient's level of physical activity, or would you be more likely to assess the patient's emotional state and discuss concurrent life events, such as work, family encounters, or special occasions? The first approach targets treatment content (ie, energy intake and expenditure), whereas the second approach focuses on the process of weight management (ie, the context in which weight loss occurs). The most successful approach involves a synthesis of these two practices. More often than not, content issues will be better addressed once process matters have been addressed.

The first step in addressing process matters is to acknowledge and respond to the patient's emotional state using open-ended, reflective statements (eg, "*It seems like* you're frustrated that you haven't lost much weight. What do you think is getting in the way?") With the information the patient provides, the health care provider can help the patient to establish a plan for behavior change. The second step is to engage the patient in the process of understanding his or her circumstance and to identify the tools necessary for building a framework that supports behavior change (eg, "You have identified a stressful situation and one activity that provides you some comfort. *What* other type of activities do you find relaxing?"). With tools in hand, the patient can construct a specific plan that will ultimately affect the content of treatment.

Advice Giving vs Problem Solving

Many providers may feel that their primary role is to give advice to patients about healthful methods of weight control. Although some education and advice is useful, most weight control patients are well aware of what they "should" eat; the problem is doing so in an environment that encourages otherwise. Therefore, an emphasis on asking questions to clarify barriers and the patient's situation is more effective than giving advice about how to "fix" the problem. A focus on problem-solving (see Part B of Chapter 9: Weight-Loss Maintenance) can model skills for patients and increase their ability to solve problems independently. Such an approach is more useful than being dependent on expert advice. As a rough indicator, the more a clinician speaks during the session, the less effective the session will be for the patient. If the clinician is talking more than 50% of the session, it is important to re-assess the balance between advice giving and problem solving.

Assessing Readiness

The trans-theoretical model of behavior change has been used as a method of determining readiness to change in a variety of health-related behaviors, such as smoking cessation (11,12). This model suggests that (1) individuals pass through three levels of readiness before actually making a change (ie, precontemplation [not considering change], contemplation [considering change], and action [making a change]), and (2) the provider's recommendations reflect the patient's readiness. There are few data to support that this model predicts obesity treatment outcome, perhaps because the constellation of behaviors required to manage weight is quite complex. Although it is useful to conceptualize stages of change, it is important to avoid the use of hard and fast categories. Unfortunately, there are no strong pretreatment predictors of outcome, other than initial weight and weight loss during the first 4 weeks of treatment (13). Therefore, clinical predictions about which patients will do well in treatment should not be made with great confidence. The five questions that follow are designed to assess "readiness" and to provide the patient and clinician with an assessment of behavioral facilitators and barriers.

Five Important Questions

Question 1: "Why Now?" (Driving force).   Why has the patient decided to lose weight at this time? Why not 6 months ago or 6 months from now? Is it because of an upcoming high school reunion or has a family member just experienced a heart attack? Whatever the reason, it will provide some insight into the patient's decision to make changes at this time.

Provider: Pat, it sounds like you've been frustrated with your weight for a long time but haven't seriously attempted to lose weight. Why have you decided to give it a try now?

Patient: Well, I know that I would be healthier if I take some weight off, but more importantly, I feel like it's time for a change. I mean, I just want to make a fresh start.

Provider: A fresh start? Tell me more about that.

Patient: Actually, I'm going through a divorce right now. I just want to leave my old life behind and start over. If I lose weight, I think I will feel more confident about myself and be willing to try things that I was scared to try before.

Question 2: "What Changes Will You Have to Make?" (Costs).   Assessing the perceived costs of weight loss can help identify any unrealistic expectations ("I need to eat less than 1,000 calories to lose weight"; "All I have to do is exercise more."). It also begins the process of having patients think through what changes need to be made and their associated costs (eg, making time for physical activity, keeping food records).

Provider: What changes do you think you'll have to make in order to lose weight?

Patient: I guess I'd have to eat less and eat better.

Provider: What does it mean to "eat less and better"?

Patient: Mainly, not eating as frequently at fast food restaurants.

Provider: What would you have to change to do that?

Patient: I guess I'd have to start preparing healthier food at home more often. I'd have to go to the grocery store more frequently than I do now, buy healthy foods, and take time out of my busy schedule to cook.

Provider: How difficult will it be for you to make these changes?

Patient: It'll be hard because I really don't have much time during the week to go to the grocery store, and I really don't know how to cook very well.

Provider: Sounds like we need to think through some solutions to these barriers, such as adjusting your schedule to make more time for you.

Question 3: "What Will Change If You Lose Weight?" (Benefits).
Discuss what positive changes patients expect after weight loss. Comparing
these to the expected costs of weight loss provides a useful assessment of motivation. If the ratio of benefits to costs is high, motivation will be high. If
the ratio is low, motivation will be low. The clinical challenge is to remove
perceived and real barriers, to make a more favorable benefit-to-cost ratio.
In addition, discussing expected benefits helps distinguish realistic ("I'll be
able to wear smaller clothes"; "I'll improve my stamina") from unrealistic
("My whole life will change"; "People will like me more") outcomes.

Provider: What do you think will change if you lose weight?
Patient: I want to fit into smaller, more stylish clothes. I want to start
dating again.
Provider: Anything else?
Patient: I'll feel better about myself, and I'll try things that I was
scared to try before.
Provider: Like what?
Patient: I would like to go back to school and take some classes so I
can pursue a career in journalism. I also love to dance, but I have
been reluctant to get out on the dance floor because of my
weight.
Provider: I wonder if you could do those things now, before you lost
weight?
Patient: Maybe I could.
Provider: When you think about the costs of losing weight (shopping, preparing food, changing your schedule) compared to the
benefits (wearing smaller sizes, dating, feeling more comfortable
with yourself) how do they compare?

*Question 4: "What Do Others Think About Your Weight?" (Social
Support).* Family, friends, and coworkers may have a variety of feelings
(ranging from empathy to hostility to jealousy) regarding another's weight
management. It is useful to explore (from a patient's perspective) specific
things that significant others do to help or hinder weight control efforts.
By knowing the patient's social support situation, the health care provider
can help the patient plan methods to identify, request, and provide feedback to others about supportive or nonsupportive behaviors. This high-
lights the need for patients to become responsible for getting the help they
need.

Provider: What do people who are close to you think about your
weight? Are there things they do to help or hinder your weight
control efforts?

Patient: I am very close to my family. I know they are all concerned about my health. My mom usually doesn't say much about my weight because she doesn't want to hurt my feelings, but I can see the look of concern when she notices that I've gained a few pounds. But at the same time, she always offers me food when I visit. My sister is thin and is happy that I've decided to lose weight, but she eats lots of junk food around me. I've gained 5 pounds since we moved in together because the junk food is lying all around the house, and I can't resist the temptation when I feel stressed, which seems to be a lot lately.

Provider: It sounds like your family is supportive of your efforts to lose weight, but may unintentionally hinder your efforts at times. What could they do or not do to make it easier for you?

Question 5: "What Else Is Going on in Your Life?" (Life Stressors). Weight control is tough work when things are going well; it is even tougher when coupled with significant life stressors, such as a job change, financial problems, or a major family illness. The health care provider can help the patient determine whether it is a favorable time to lose weight or whether it is more realistic to prevent further weight gain at this time. The decision is ultimately the patient's. The role of the health care provider is to assist patients in making feasible dietary and activity changes in the context of the patient's current situation.

Provider: During our conversation you mentioned two major changes that have recently occurred in your life—a divorce and moving in with your sister. Is there anything else going on in your life?

Patient: No, not really . . . just the usual job pressures.

Provider: Tell me a little bit more about why you decided to move in with your sister.

Patient: Well, part of the reason is because I feel like I could use some emotional support during the divorce procedures. I'm also having some financial difficulties and it really helps to share the rent with somebody.

Provider: It seems like you have a lot going on right now. Do you think it's the best time to take on a major weight loss effort?

Patient: I really want to make some positive changes in my life. There is a lot going on that I cannot completely control, but I feel that weight loss is one area where I can have some control.

Provider: The decision is yours to make. Although weight control is a positive stressor, it is a stressor nonetheless. We'll have to watch for any effects that your weight control efforts have on your other stressors and vice versa as we go through the process. Weight loss is difficult, but it is possible. You can count on me to help.

Adherence

Improving Adherence

Several straightforward guidelines can help patients improve their adherence to the behaviors necessary for effective weight control. They are discussed below.

- *Be clear that the patient knows the rationale for changing behavior (WHY).* It is important to ensure that patients understand the rationale for a specific behavior change. Questions such as "Why do you think I'm asking you to keep food records? Have you found them useful in the past?" will clarify whether the patient sees any value in record keeping. Patients are adult learners who need to be engaged in the process of behavior change. Simply telling them that "it is important" or "good for them" does not suffice.
- *Identify a goal and establish a specific plan (WHAT).* Short-term goals should be based on behavior rather than weight, because many factors other than behavior (salt, fluid, humidity) affect weight in the short term. When helping patients select goals, it is important to describe the behavior in concrete and specific terms: Help patients select a specific plan (eg, limit eating to 300 kcal between 7:00 PM and 10:00 PM or walk for 20 minutes after dinner on Monday, Wednesday, and Friday) rather than a general platitude (eg, eat less at night or exercise more). The more specific the goal, the better.
- *Identify facilitators and barriers to success (HOW).* To successfully execute the plan, the process must be thought through from beginning to end. It is rare that any plan will proceed without an occasional glitch; therefore, it is important to help patients think through the steps that will be necessary to achieve their goal (eg, purchasing alternative foods for evening consumption or having a spouse help with household duties after dinner), including steps to avoid or overcome potential barriers.
- *Follow-up at the next visit.* Have the patient make a written record of the plan and key steps in its implementation. In addition, make a brief note in the chart documenting the specific plan. At the next visit, review the patient's progress with the specific plan, rather than asking generally, "How did it go?" Was the behavior accomplished or not? If successful, what strategies did the patient use to achieve the goal? If unsuccessful, what things got in the way, and how can they be removed in the future?

Patients benefit more from examining *how* behavior changed or did not change than from focusing on *why* things did not go as planned.

Dealing With Nonadherence

In an ideal world, the steps described above would reliably produce adherence, weight loss, and satisfied patients and practitioners. The reality is that effective weight control is a learned skill. Like the development of any other skill, setbacks are to be expected. Effectively managing nonadherence is an essential skill for both patients and practitioners. The following suggestions are designed to help the health care provider and the patient deal with nonadherence.

- *Assume that a lack of planning or skills rather than a lack of motivation is the reason for nonadherence.* When things do not go as planned, it is important to focus on what can be done differently in terms of planning or coping skills. This emphasizes a plan of action rather than fruitless discussions about motivation. Motivation (the ratio of benefits to costs) can be addressed after multiple attempts at planning and skill building have faltered, but the first assumption should be that skills, rather than motivation, need to be enhanced.
- *Analyze what happened and how it can be prevented in the future.* Cast setbacks as an opportunity to refine weight control skills. Ask enough questions to understand HOW things did not go as planned (eg, time, place, activity, emotions, or the sequence of events). What specifically got in the way and how can it be removed? Instilling hope is an essential feature of an effective therapeutic relationship. Having patients think through how they would deal with the same situation in the future will increase self-efficacy and give hope.
- *Help patients recognize nonadherence and assume responsibility for their actions.* Patients may attribute nonadherence to factors that are beyond their control (eg, people or activities). Identifying behaviors that can be managed not only empowers the patient; it also underscores that the patient is responsible for problem solving.
- *Avoid criticizing patients.* Weight control is tough work and patients need to know that you will not give up on them. Criticizing patients or questioning their motivation does little for improving adherence and has adverse effects on the patient-provider relationship. Patients will struggle, and they need to know that your support is unconditional.
- *Preserve the patient's self-esteem and be patient.* Realize that patients often feel frustrated and discouraged when they have not followed their intended plan. Feelings of failure are likely to occur when one expects to achieve perfection. Identifying small and positive accomplishments and

pointing out that the goal is not to achieve perfection will help boost morale and self-esteem. Both the health care provider and the patient should keep in mind that long-term changes do not occur overnight.

- *Share your frustration with colleagues, so it does not affect your work with patients.* Treating refractory conditions like obesity can undermine your own professional self-esteem. Read the scientific literature regularly to be reassured that no one has yet cured obesity! Discussing frustrations with colleagues can have positive therapeutic benefits and can reduce the potential for burnout and ineffective patient care.

Common Clinical Challenges

Nonadherence to Food Records

The importance of keeping food records for short- and long-term weight control is well established (14). It is just as well established that adherence to self-monitoring is less than optimal at times. Several suggestions for addressing this common occurrence are described below.

- *Assess benefits.* The first step is to assess whether patients perceive any benefit to keeping food records. (When you do keep records, do you find them useful?) If there is no perceived benefit, attempts at improving adherence will be undermined.
- *Identify barriers.* Open-ended questions, such as "Tell me about what gets in the way when you try to keep food records" or "What changes do you think you'll have to make in order to keep food records," may help clarify barriers and underscore areas for problem solving.
- *Make it easier to be successful.* Small successes lead to bigger successes. Rather than insisting on a 7-day food record, it may be a better first step to keep a 3-day record or simply to record at high-risk times (between dinner and bedtime). Consider also shortening the assessment period. Instead of waiting until the next scheduled appointment, the provider may want to call the patient at a specified time to assess progress with record keeping in a few days.

Plateaus

Inevitably, weight loss slows or stops. Predictably, fears and frustrations are common at this time. It is worthwhile for patients and health care providers to pause and examine the situation.

- *Accept the facts.* Weight loss tends to slow down after the initial 4 to 6 months. The degree to which this is due to behavioral (decreased adherence) or biological (body-weight regulation) causes is unknown (15).

What is clear is that fewer calories are required to support a smaller body. So, the same energy intake that produced weight loss at 220 lb will produce less weight loss at 200 lb. Thus, a slowing of weight loss is to be expected, even if patients remain significantly overweight.

- *Assess dietary and activity patterns.* Whether the plateau is behavioral, biological, or both, it is important to assess diet and activity patterns. It may be that record keeping has become less frequent or accurate or that overall adherence is more difficult after an initial significant (10%) weight loss. It is tough work to continually monitor behaviors, and the distress about weight is likely to be diminished after an initial weight loss.
- *Make a plan.* If adherence is diminished, discuss the realities of chronic care and help patients make small changes that will affect energy balance. This is not the time to set goals as if it were the first week of treatment. If adherence seems adequate, it may be time to do the hard work of maintaining weight for a few months, to collect information on how difficult that process is. After a few months, the patient can decide whether or not to pursue additional weight loss.

Unrealistic Expectations

One of the greatest challenges in the clinical management of obese patients is addressing the significant disparity between actual and expected weight losses. Although professionals generally accept a 10% weight loss as successful (based on the associated improvements in comorbidities), patients typically seek weight losses that approximate 30% reductions in body weight (16,17). Several recommendations may help patients to accept more modest weight loss outcomes as successful.

- *Be clear about what weight loss does and does not.* Weight loss will make you healthier, but it does not guarantee a better job, a happier marriage, or other things that many patients seek through weight loss. Discussing (before treatment) what else patients expect to change besides their weight will help to identify any unrealistic expectations or magical thinking regarding weight loss (See section on assessing readiness, earlier in this chapter).
- *Focus on nonweight outcomes.* Focus on the many *nonweight* changes, such as improvements in serum lipids, blood pressure, and glycemic control. In addition, prompt patients to assess changes in their quality of life, such as increased energy, being able to keep up with children or grandchildren, and climbing stairs without shortness of breath.
- *Discuss biological limits.* In short, acknowledge what patients already know: not everyone who eats the same and exercises the same weighs the

same. Weight is not infinitely malleable, and there are likely biological boundaries that set limits for weight loss. Help patients to focus on behavioral changes that improve health and to worry less about the ultimate number of pounds lost. Patients will need your help to counter the cultural myth that "you can weigh whatever you want."

To Diet or Not To Diet?

During the last 15 years, dieting has come under attack by a growing movement that contends that "diets don't work" and that their physical and psychological ill effects far outweigh any fleeting benefits (18). This movement, often referred to as "anti-dieting" or "undieting," has gained support from professionals and nonprofessionals alike. The growing discontent with dieting and a search for alternative approaches is based on three premises: (1) dieting confers a host of harmful physical and psychological effects, (2) dieting does not result in sustained weight loss, and (3) basic assumptions about the causes and consequences of overweight are incorrect. In general, these approaches suggest that overweight persons give up dieting and accept themselves as they are.

Undieting approaches differ in their specific methods, but all approaches generally seek to (1) increase awareness about dieting's ill effects; (2) encourage the use of internal cues, such as hunger and fullness, rather than external cues, such as calories or fat grams, to guide eating behavior; (3) enhance knowledge about the biological basis of body weight; (4) improve self-esteem and body image through self-acceptance rather than weight loss; and (5) increase physical activity. Most of the early studies on undieting programs were descriptive in nature. These studies were helpful in collecting initial data about novel approaches, but they provided no comparisons with traditional dieting approaches. More recent controlled studies showed minimal weight loss but significant improvements in body image and self-esteem (18).

Strengths

A major strength of the undieting movement is its continued emphasis on the long-term ineffectiveness of dieting. Although increased physical activity and continued patient-practitioner contact after treatment significantly improve the maintenance of weight loss in the year after treatment (see Chapter 9: Weight-Loss Maintenance), weight regain is the most frequent long-term outcome of dieting. Clearly, there is a need for new approaches that are not based on dieting. The anti-dieting movement has provided one such alternative.

Perhaps the greatest strength of the undieting movement is the affirmation of a person's worth, no matter what he or she weighs. The message is so counterculture that it can seem ridiculous to suggest that overweight persons should like themselves or that overweight does not result from a lack of character or willpower. Such stereotypes are not only inaccurate; they are cruel. Like other forms of discrimination and prejudice, they should not be tolerated.

Weaknesses

The most significant weakness of the undieting approaches is the lack of scientific support. It is troubling that the number of undieting books increases daily, although few controlled studies demonstrate their effectiveness. No approach, no matter how well intentioned or sensible, should be touted as a superior alternative to dieting without data. Claims of "health at any size" need to be supported by studies that measure changes in fitness, serum lipoproteins, glycemic control, and other cardiovascular risk factors before and after nondieting interventions. Unfortunately, the significant increase of anti-dieting books, videos, and tapes makes it difficult to distinguish these approaches from the multitude of new diet books that are also published without scientific evaluation. Obese patients deserve better. They are entitled to know the short- and long-term results of alternative treatments, so that they can make informed decisions about their health and weight.

The development of undieting approaches represents an exciting development in the care of overweight and obese persons. These approaches should be carefully evaluated before being widely disseminated. Such information will help overweight persons make informed decisions about managing their health and weight. Whether the resolution ultimately is to diet or not to diet, we hope that professionals can help overweight persons realize that weight is just one factor that describes them—yet it does not define them.

Final Note

Health care providers can provide a great service to obese patients by reminding them that their worth is not measured on the scale. Patients should be encouraged to take themselves, their health, and thus their weight seriously, rather than attempting to lose weight so that they can like themselves. Reaffirming the patient's self-worth, independent of body weight, is perhaps one of the most powerful interventions a practitioner can provide an obese patient. As Stunkard suggests, "As with any chronic illness, we rarely have an opportunity to cure, but we do have an opportunity to treat the patient with respect. Such an experience may be the greatest gift that [we] can give an obese patient" (9).

References

1. Stunkard AJ, Sobal J. Psychosocial consequences of obesity. In: Brownell KD, Fairburn CG, eds. *Eating Disorders and Obesity: A Comprehensive Handbook*. New York, NY: Guilford Press, 1995:417–421.
2. Price JH, Desmond SM, Krol RA, Snyder FF, O'Connell JK. Family practice physicians' beliefs, attitudes, and practices regarding obesity. *Am J Prev Med*. 1987;3:339–345.
3. Foster GD, Wadden TA, Makris A, Davidson D, Sanderson RS, Allison DA, Kessler A. Primary care physicians' attitudes about obesity and its treatment. *Obes Res*. In press.
4. Maiman LA, Wang VL, Becker MH, Finlay J, Simonson M. Attitudes toward obesity and the obese among professionals. *J Am Diet Assoc*. 1979;74:331–336.
5. Oberrieder H, Walker R, Monroe D, Adeyanju M. Attitudes of dietetics students and registered dietitians toward obesity. *J Am Diet Assoc*. 1995;95:914–916.
6. McArthur L, Ross J. Attitudes of registered dietitians toward personal overweight and overweight clients. *J Am Diet Assoc*. 1997;97:63–66.
7. Puhl R, Brownell KD. Bias, discrimination, and obesity. *Obes Res*. 2001;9:788–805.
8. Foster GD. Goals and strategies to improve behavior change effectiveness. In: Bessesen DH, Kushner RF, eds. *Evaluation and Management of Obesity*. Philadelphia, Pa: Hanley & Belfus; 2002:29–32.
9. Stunkard AJ. Talking with patients. In: Stunkard AJ, Wadden TA, eds. *Obesity: Theory and Therapy*. 2nd ed. New York, NY: Raven Press; 1993:355–363.
10. Laquatra I, Danish S. Counseling skills for behavior change. In: King KK, Klawitter B, eds. *Nutrition Therapy: Advanced Counseling Skills*. Lake Dallas, Tex: Helm Seminars; 1995:123–134.
11. Prochaska J, Johnson S, Lee P. The trans-theoretical model of behavior change. In: Shumaker SA, Schron EB, Ockene JK, eds. *The Handbook of Behavior Change*. 2nd ed. New York, NY: Springer Publishing; 1998:59–84.
12. Prochaska J, DiClemente C. Stages and processes of self-change of smoking: toward an integrative model of change. *J Consult Clin Psychol*. 1983;51:390–395.
13. Wadden TA, Letizia KA. Predictors of attrition and outcome. In: Wadden TA, Stunkard AJ, eds. *Obesity: Theory and Therapy*. New York, NY: Raven Press; 1993:197–218.
14. O'Neil, PM. Assessing dietary intake in the management of obesity. *Obes Res*. 2001;9(Suppl 5):S361–S366.
15. Korner J, Aronne LJ. The emerging science of body weight regulation and its impact on obesity treatment. *J Clin Invest*. 2003;111:565–570.

16. Foster GD, Wadden TA, Vogt RA, Brewer G. What is a reasonable weight loss? Patients' expectations and evaluations of obesity treatment. *J Consult Clin Psychol*. 1997;65:79–85.

17. Foster GD, Wadden TA, Phelan S, Sarwer DB, Swain Sanderson R. Obese patients' perceptions of treatment outcomes and the factors that influence them. *Arch Intern Med*. 2001;161:2133–2139.

18. Foster GD, McGuckin B. Nondieting approaches: principles, practices, and evidence. In: Wadden TA, Stunkard AJ, eds. *Handbook of Obesity*. New York, NY: Guilford Press; 1993:506–512.

Chapter 5

Dietary Approaches

PART A. Overview

Eileen Kennedy, DSc, RD

The Best Diet?

The fact that there are more than 1,200 "weight-loss" books on the market underscores society's quest for the perfect diet. Approximately 90% have been published since 1997 (1). The answer to the "best" diet question is, of course, not simple and depends on individual factors (eg, health conditions, age) and goals (eg, weight loss, weight maintenance, improvement of medical conditions). By the time overweight or obese patients see a professional for advice, they may already have strong preconceived notions about "what works" for weight loss and/or may be very disillusioned. It is useful, then, to be aware of the benefits and liabilities of various dietary approaches to weight loss. The purpose of this overview is to summarize the research on diets used for weight management and to identify gaps in our knowledge.

Types of Diets

When trying to understand the effects of various dietary approaches to weight management, it is useful to think of categories based on macronutrient composition. Despite the enormous number of diets and diet books available, most fall into three main categories.

- *Low-Carbohydrate, High-Fat Diet*—Defined as <20% of total energy from carbohydrate or <100 g of total carbohydrate. Diets such as the Atkins diet and Protein Power would fall into this category.
- *Very-Low-Fat, High-Carbohydrate Diet*—Defined as ≤10% of total energy from fat and >55% of energy from carbohydrate. Low-fat and very-low-fat diets were originally developed for individuals with heart disease. Only recently have they become popular for weight loss. Low-fat and very-low-fat diets that are high in complex carbohydrates, fruits, and vegetables are naturally high in fiber and low in energy density. Programs such as Dean Ornish's Program for Reversing Heart Disease and Nathan Pritikin's Program would fall into this category.
- *Moderate-Fat, High-Carbohydrate Diet*—Defined as between 20% and 30% of total energy from fat and >55% of energy from carbohydrate. Diets such as the American Heart Association's Shape Up America and many of the commercial weight-loss programs (such as Weight Watchers and Jenny Craig) would fall into this category.

Weight Loss

Short-term Weight Loss

There is an enormous body of literature on weight-reduction diets, which dates back to the 1930s. A review of more than 200 research studies on diet and weight loss conducted during the past 60 years indicates that any diet that reduces caloric intake will result in weight loss (1), regardless of the macronutrient content (fat, protein, or carbohydrate). Analysis of sample menus from all these categories of diets reveal energy intakes of 1,200 to 1,600 kcal (1). For most overweight and obese persons, these energy prescriptions will result in an energy deficit and weight loss. In sum, all popular diets, as well as diets recommended by governmental organizations, will result in weight loss if specific dietary guidelines are followed. Regardless of macronutrient composition, low-carbohydrate diets or moderate-, low-, or very-low-fat diets typically produce weight loss in the range of 6% to 10% of baseline weight over a 3- to 6-month period (2–9). However, average weight loss can be quite variable within the study population (1). Reasons for this variability are not entirely known but may relate to variations in compliance with the reduction diet.

Some authors in the popular literature suggest that there is a "metabolic advantage" in following a low-carbohydrate, high-fat diet and that calories do not matter (10). Developers of low-carbohydrate diets claim that people can eat a greater number of calories and still lose weight. There is, however, no evidence in the scientific literature that supports this claim.

Studies have determined that individuals who consume a low-carbohydrate diet lose weight because they are eating fewer calories (11–16).

Long-term Weight Loss

The consistency of short-term weight loss across dietary approaches is matched by the lack of long-term success across modalities (see Chapter 9: Weight-Loss Maintenance). Low-fat, high-carbohydrate approaches are the most researched. Approximately one third of the weight lost is regained in the year after treatment; two thirds is regained at 3 years; and virtually all weight is regained at 5 years (Chapter 9: Weight-Loss Maintenance). In the only study of a low-carbohydrate diet lasting longer than 6 months, weight was regained between 6 and 12 months (17), making it no different at 1 year from a low-calorie, moderate-fat, high-carbohydrate approach. Longer-term data for these types of popular diets are not available, making any conclusions about long-term efficacy of low-carbohydrate approaches impossible. There are, however, longer-term data available on other popular diets. Ornish et al (9,18), report successful 1- and 5-year follow-up data for individuals eating a very-low-fat diet. Fletchner-Mors et al (19) reported successful 4-year maintenance data for SlimFast, and Heshka et al (20) compared self-help with Weight Watchers over 2 years and found a structured weight-control program more successful in managing overweight.

Nutritional Adequacy

No single food can supply all the nutrients needed by the human body. Data from a nationally representative sample of the US adult population show that individuals who eat foods from all the major food groups are significantly more likely to consume a nutritionally adequate diet (21). Low-carbohydrate, high-fat diets are inadequate in a range of nutrients, including vitamin E, vitamin A, thiamin, vitamin B-6, folate, calcium, magnesium, iron, zinc, potassium, and dietary fiber (1). A dietary supplement should be routinely recommended for people on high-fat, low-carbohydrate diets.

Analyses of suggested menus for very-low-fat diet plans indicate that they are deficient in vitamin E, B-12, and zinc. Because very-low-fat diet plans contain almost no animal protein, it is not surprising that B-12 intakes would be low. In addition, given the low level of total fat in these diet plans, vitamin E levels are low. A dietary supplement should be recommended as part of the very-low-fat diet regimen. Because the moderate-fat, high-carbohydrate diet has a variety of healthy food choices, it is the most nutritionally adequate (1).

Hunger and Compliance

Dietary compliance is a function of many factors—nutritional, psychological, social, and biochemical. Diet type may not be the most important element in long-term compliance to a weight-loss diet. Fat-restricted diets (both low-fat and moderate-fat) have been shown to produce a high degree of satiety (19,22–24). People who consumed fat-reduced diets were less likely to complain of hunger and commented on "too much food" (25) compared with their typical baseline diet. This is, in large part, due to the fact that reduced-fat diets tend to have a low-energy density, and a greater physical quantity of food can be consumed at a lower caloric intake.

Metabolic Effects

Any diet that results in energy restriction and weight loss improves the metabolic profile of the individual. Reduction of energy intake, regardless of the macronutrient content, improves glycemic control (26–28). As body weight decreases, there is a concurrent drop in blood insulin levels.

Low-carbohydrate, high-fat, high-protein diets are ketogenic. The ketosis produced on low-carbohydrate diets can cause significant increases in

---

What We Know

- Weight loss is independent of diet composition. Caloric balance is the major determinant of weight loss. Diets that reduce energy intake result in weight loss.
- Weight loss, regardless of the macronutrient composition of the diet, produces metabolic changes, including improved glycemic control, decreased blood lipids, and decreased blood pressure. The magnitude of these may vary by type of diet and amount of weight loss.
- The amount of weight loss is variable and tends to decline with the length of the study.

What We Don't Know

- The long-term metabolic effects of different diet types on bone changes, renal function, and lipoprotein profile, once the weight-loss phase has ended.
- How to increase adherence to the dietary regimen long-term. (This will be discussed in detail in Chapter 9: Weight-Loss Maintenance).
- Whether effects of different weight-loss diet types on health status differ depending on body mass index.

the blood uric acid concentration. Other effects of low-carbohydrate diets include decreased blood glucose, decreased serum insulin levels, decreased total cholesterol and LDL-C, and decreased blood pressure (29–31).

Moderate-fat-reduction diets also have associated metabolic effects, including decreased total cholesterol and LDL-C, decreased serum insulin, and reduced blood pressure (26). Similarly, the metabolic effects of low-fat and very-low-fat diets include reduced total cholesterol and LDL-C, decreased serum insulin, and decreased blood pressure (32–34). Some study results have raised concerns that very-low-fat, high-carbohydrate diets raise triglyceride levels and lower HDL-C (35–37).

Weight loss, regardless of diet type, results in an improved lipid profile. Total cholesterol, LDL-C, HDL-C, and triglycerides decrease as body weight decreases (38). Three recent, randomized research studies provide some intriguing findings on low-carbohydrate, high-fat diets for periods of 6 months (39,40) and 1 year (17). In all three studies, people on the low-carbohydrate diets lost significantly more weight during the first 6 months than individuals on low-fat, high-carbohydrate diets. However, the differences in weight loss were not significant at 1 year (17). In addition, the low-carbohydrate diet produced increases in HDL-C (17) and decreases in serum triglycerides (17,37,39).

References

1. Freedman MR, King J, Kennedy E. Popular diets: a scientific review. *Obes Res*. 2001;9(Suppl 1):1S–40S.
2. Worthington BS, Taylor LE. Balanced low-calorie vs high-protein, low-carbo-hydrate reducing diets. I. Weight loss, nutrient intake, and subjective evalua-tion. *J Am Diet Assoc*. 1974;64:47–51.
3. Rabast U, Kasper H, Schonborn J. Comparative studies in obese subjects fed carbohydrate-restricted and high-carbohydrate 1,000-calorie formula diets. *Nutr Metab*. 1978;22:269–277.
4. Baron JA, Schori A, Crow B, Carter R, Mann JI. A randomized controlled trial of low-carbohydrate and low-fat/high-fiber diets for weight loss. *Am J Public Health*. 1986;76:1293–1296.
5. Buzzard IM, Asp EH, Chlebowski RT, Boyar AP, Jeffery RW, Nixon DW, Blackburn GL, Jochimsen PR, Scanlon EF, Insull W Jr. Diet intervention meth-ods to reduce fat intake: nutrient and food group composition of self-selected low-fat diets. *J Am Diet Assoc*. 1990;90:42–50, 53.
6. Hammer RL, Barrier CA, Roundy ES, Bradford JM, Fisher AG. Calorie-restricted low-fat diet and exercise in obese women. *Am J Clin Nutr*. 1989; 49:77–85.
7. Schlundt DG, Hill JO, Pope-Cordle J, Arnold D, Vitrs K, Katahn M. Random-ized evaluation of a low-fat ad libitum carbohydrate diet for weight reduction. *Int J Obes Relat Metab Disord*. 1993;17:623–629.

8. Djuric Z, Uhley VE, Depper JB, Brooks KM, Lababidi S, Heilbrun LK. A clinical trial to selectively change dietary fat and/or energy intake in women: the Women's Diet Study. *Nutr Cancer.* 1999:3427–3435.

9. Ornish D, Brown SE, Scherwitz LW, Billings JH, Armstrong WT, Ports TA, McLanahan SM, Kirkeeide RL, Brand RJ, Gould KL. Can lifestyle changes reverse coronary heart disease? *Lancet.* 1990;336:129–133.

10. Atkins RC. *Dr. Atkins' New Diet Revolution.* New York, NY: Avon Books; 1992.

11. Evans E, Stock AL, Yudkin J. The absence of undesirable changes during consumption of the low-carbohydrate diet. *Nutr Metab.* 1974;17:360–367.

12. Yudkin J, Carey M. The treatment of obesity by the "high-fat" diet: the inevitability of calories. *Lancet.* 1960;2:939

13. Rickman F, Mitchell N, Dingman J, Dalen JE. Changes in serum cholesterol during the Stillman diet. *JAMA.* 1974;228:54–58.

14. Larosa JC, Gordon A, Muesing R, Rosing DR. Effects of high-protein, low-carbohydrate dieting on plasma lipoproteins and body weight. *J Am Diet Assoc.* 1980;77:264–270.

15. Westman EC, Yancy WS, Edman JS, Tomlin KF, Perkins CE. Effect of 6-month adherence to a very low-carbohydrate diet program. *Am J Med.* 2002; 113: 30–36.

16. Bravata Dena M, Sanders L, Huang J, Krumholz HM, Olkin I, Gardner CD, Bravata Dawn M. Efficacy and safety of low-carbohydrate diets: a systematic review. *JAMA.* 2003;289:1837–1850.

17. Foster GD, Wyatt HR, Hill JO, McGuckin BG, Brill C, Mohammed BS, Szapary PO, Rader DJ, Edman JS, Klein S. A randomized trial of a low-carbohydrate diet for obesity. *N Engl J Med.* 2003;348:2082–2090.

18. Ornish D, Scherwitz LW, Billings JH, Brown SE, Gould KL, Merritt TA, Sparler S, Armstrong WT, Ports TA, Kirkeeide RL, Hogeboom C, Brand RJ. Intensive lifestyle changes for reversal of coronary heart disease. *JAMA.* 1998;280: 2001–2007.

19. Fletchner-Mors M, Ditschuneit HH, Johnson TD, Suchard MA, Adler G. Metabolic and weight-loss effects of long-term dietary intervention in obese patients: four-year results. *Obes Res.* 2000;8:399–402.

20. Heshka S, Anderson JW, Atkinson RL, Greenway FL, Hill JO, Phinney SD, Kolotkin RL, Miller-Kovach K, Pi-Sunyer FX. Weight loss with self-help compared with a structured commercial program: a randomized trial. *JAMA.* 2003;289:1792–1798.

21. Kennedy ET, Bowman SA, Spence JT, Freedman M, King J. Popular diets: correlation to health, nutrition, and obesity. *J Am Diet Assoc.* 2001;101:411–420.

22. Blundell JE, Green S, Burley V. Carbohydrates and human appetite. *Am J Clin Nutr.* 1994;59:728S–734S.

23. Rolls BJ. The role of energy density in the overconsumption of fat. *J Nutr.* 2000;130(2S Suppl):268S–271S.

24. Kendall A, Levitsky DA, Strupp BJ, Lissner L. Weight loss on a low-fat diet: consequence of the imprecision of the control of food intake in humans. *Am J Clin Nutr.* 1991;53:1124–1129.

25. Schaefer EJ, Lichtenstein AH, Lamon-Fava S, McNamara JR, Schaefer MM, Rasmussen H, Ordovas JM. Body weight and low-density lipoprotein cholesterol changes after consumption of a low-fat ad libitum diet. *JAMA*. 1995; 274:1450–1455.
26. Golay A, Allaz AF, Morel Y, de Tonnac N, Tankova S, Reaven GM. Similar weight loss with low- or high-carbohydrate diets. *Am J Clin Nutr*. 1996;63: 174–178.
27. Grey N, Kipnis DM. Effect of diet composition on the hyperinsulinemia of obesity. *N Engl J Med*. 1971;285:827-831.
28. Heilbronn LK, Noakes M, Clifton PM. Effect of energy restriction, weight loss, and diet composition on plasma lipids and glucose in patients with type 2 diabetes. *Diabetes Care*. 1999;22:889–895.
29. Alford BB, Blankenship AC, Hagen RD. The effects of variations in carbohydrate, protein, and fat content of the diet upon weight loss, blood values, and nutrient intake of adult obese women. *J Am Diet Assoc*. 1990;90:534–540.
30. Lewis SB, Wallin JD, Kane JP, Gerich JE. Effect of diet composition on metabolic adaptations to hypocaloric nutrition: comparison of high-carbohydrate and high-fat isocaloric diets. *Am J Clin Nutr*. 1977;30:160–170.
31. Krehl WA, Lopez-SA, Good EI, Hodges RE. Some metabolic changes induced by low-carbohydrate diets. *Am J Clin Nutr*. 1967;20:139–148.
32. Ornish D. Avoiding revascularization with lifestyle changes: the Multicenter Lifestyle Demonstration Project. *Am J Cardiol*. 1998;82:72T–76T.
33. Boyar AP, Rose DP, Loughridge JR, Engle A, Palgi A, Laakso K, Kinne D, Wynder EL. Response to a diet low in total fat in women with post-menopausal breast cancer: a pilot study. *Nutr Cancer*. 1988;11:93–99.
34. Barnard RJ. Effects of life-style modification on serum lipids. *Arch Intern Med*. 1991;151:1389–1394.
35. Noakes M, Clifton PM. Changes in plasma lipids and other cardiovascular risk factors during 3 energy-restricted diets differing in total fat and fatty acid composition. *Am J Clin Nutr*. 2000;71:706–712.
36. Lichtenstein AH, Van Horn L. AHA Science Advisory. Very-low-fat diets. *Circulation*. 1998;98:935–939.
37. Surwit RS, Feinglos MN, McCaskill CC, Clay SL, Babyak MA, Brownlow BS, Plaisted CS, Lin PH. Metabolic and behavioral effects of a high-sucrose diet during weight loss. *Am J Clin Nutr*. 1997;65:908–915.
38. National Institutes of Health, National Heart, Lung, and Blood Institute. Obesity Education Initiative. Clinical guidelines on the identification, evaluation, and treatment of overweight and obesity in adults. *Obes Res*. 1998;6(Suppl 2): 51S–210S.
39. Samaha FF, Iqbal N, Seshadri P, Chicano KL, Daily DA, McGrory J, Williams T, Williams M, Gracely EJ, Stern L. A low-carbohydrate as compared with low-fat diet in severe obesity. *N Engl J Med*. 2003;348:2074–2081.
40. Brehm BJ, Seeley RJ, Daniels SR, D'Alessio DA. A randomized trial comparing a very low carbohydrate diet and a calorie-restricted low fat diet on body weight and cardiovascular risk factors in healthy women. *J Clin Endocrinol Metab*. 2003;88:1617–1623.

PART B. Practical Applications

Rebecca Reeves, PhD, RD,
Mary Pat Bolton, MA, RD, and Molly Gee, MEd, RD

A perfect dietary prescription for weight loss would be one in which the diet is complete in all nutrients but calories. In reality, most weight-loss diets are deficient in a variety of nutrients. With the seduction of popular diets that promise "magic" and "ease," preference for certain foods over others, and different cultural environments, it can be a significant challenge for the health care professional to offer advice. How do you help the overweight woman who believes her body cannot metabolize carbohydrates? Or the man who swears he can only lose weight if he does not eat during the day? What about the person who feels she has no control over her food, because her grandmother does all the cooking for the three generations who live in her house? How do you guide the client who has reached a weight plateau or the harried, working mom who is having trouble adhering to a prescribed plan? In other words, How do you help real people choose healthful weight-reduction diets that make sense in varied lifestyles? This chapter addresses the practical aspects of helping clients choose a healthful and effective diet for weight loss. Because this topic is so large and has such an abundance of ideas, the diets discussed have been chosen because they are the most topical and represent the major categories of weight-loss regimens.

Guiding Principles

Not long ago, it was customary to coax clients to follow one diet only: a well-balanced, lower-fat, moderate regimen. In the medical profession's vernacular, there was no other safe way to lose weight. In fact, it is not clear that this is so. Weight loss itself, often irrespective of the type of diet, improves the health profile (1) and losing 5% to 10% improves the clinical picture significantly (2,3).

As the epidemic of obesity in the United States grows more alarming and the health effects more apparent, there is an argument to be made for reducing weight by any means and for putting more emphasis on maintaining those losses. People are going to follow the popular diets of the moment, with or without guidance and encouragement from a health professional. The clinician may know there is no magic to these popular diets and that they are not as easy to follow as they purport to be. But the dieter does not realize that these diets, like as all diets, work simply because energy intake is reduced. Clinicians may be concerned with the potential side effects from nutrient deficiencies or unhealthy fat sources, but clients usually just want results. If these popular diets are approached with some openness by the clinician, there may be ways to design a reasonably healthful weight-loss program, even within the confines of a diet that eliminates bread, stays within the "zone," or avoids carrots because they supposedly have a high glycemic index (GI).

Some guiding principles that can help the clinician and the client come to an equitable solution follow.

1. *Flexibility*—It is often the case that the client will have a preconceived notion of what is best for him or her. As professionals, it works against us to immediately negate that notion, if that is what the client thinks will work. If initial weight loss is a strong predictor of weight loss (4), then it makes good sense to find a diet to which the client is willing to adhere.
2. *Health Status*—To ensure the best outcomes, the primary care physician must agree that the diet does not put the client at undue risk (5).
3. *Nutritional Improvement*—Small modifications can usually be made in any diet to improve nutritional content, even while adhering to the client's wishes.
4. *Big Picture*—What are the goals for the client, given his or her lifestyle? If the diet is too confining for long-term use, what are the goals after the diet? What are the criteria for success (consider health, nonbingeing, "normalizing" eating, and weight loss)?
5. *Weight Loss*—Both the client and the clinician hope the client will lose weight. However, the first diet plan may not work. Therefore, the clinician should let the client know that there are plenty of variations for any diet plan, and together they will find one that produces the desired outcome.

The following two clinical cases, involving Janice and Robert, will illustrate the guiding principles.

Case Study. Janice—Part I

Janice is a 45-year-old woman who is 65 inches tall and weighs 180 lb. Her BMI is 30, indicative of class I obesity (6). Recent lab results include serum cholesterol: 215 mg/dL; LDL-C: 134 mg/dL; HDL-C: 42mg/dL; serum triglycerides: 195 mg/dL; fasting blood glucose: 119 mg/dL; and blood pressure: 130/85.

Janice considers herself a healthy person, although she realizes that her family history of diabetes and cardiac disease may put her at some risk as she gets older. She is also concerned because her doctor told her that she has metabolic syndrome (7) and weight loss would improve her risk profile. She feels that her health is added motivation to lose weight.

Weight History

Janice has lost many pounds on popular diets, but she always regains the weight when she resumes her regular eating pattern. She had gained 15 lb after the birth of each of her two children, and in the last year she gained another 20 lb. She complains of feeling hungrier now than ever before.

Dietary Patterns

Janice has tried low-calorie, low-fat diets many times but is convinced that they do not work for her. She wants an eating plan that will curb her constant hunger, which she firmly believes is the basis of her poor eating habits. She claims that when she eats breakfast, she gets hungrier, so she drinks coffee with small amounts of artificial sweetener but has nothing else all morning long. Sometimes she misses lunch as well. Occasionally, she consumes doughnuts during meetings at the office. Further review of her eating plan indicates that she consumes few green vegetables, except for a salad when she eats at restaurants. Her fruit intake consists of orange juice a couple of times each week or one piece of fruit, and she consumes few grain products that are high in fiber.

Janice lives with her husband and teenage sons, all of whom are in good health and not overweight. She keeps chips, ice cream, soft drinks, cookies, and pizza on hand. She makes a full dinner when she gets home, usually meat or chicken, rice, potatoes, a cooked vegetable, salad, and rolls. If she is especially hungry, she may snack on cheese and crackers while she prepares the meal. Between dinner and bedtime, she watches television, going back and forth into the kitchen to get tea or a snack. Sometimes she will nibble on crackers or fat-free frozen yogurt. Sometimes she will eat her family's cookies.

The Diet Request

Because of her intense hunger, she thinks a low-carbohydrate or low-GI diet would be appropriate. She is afraid that she is allergic to carbohydrates or that her insulin is not working properly and that she needs to stay away from carbohydrates forever. Although she says that she wants to stop "dieting" and make eating changes that will allow her to lose her weight and maintain it, she's tired of "wearing" 50 extra pounds and wants it off now.

The Professional's Dilemma

The diet that Janice is requesting has to be addressed first. In reality, Janice is suggesting two different diets: an Atkins type (8) and a glycemic type (9). If she has been reading about the glycemic diet but her neighbor lost weight on the Atkins, which one is she more interested in trying first? The clinician needs to explain the diets and the pitfalls of both.

Carbohydrate-Restricted Diets

Carbohydrate-restricted diets tend to be <100 g of carbohydrate per day and purport to cause ketosis (10), even though the level of ketosis is quite small, if at all (11). Popular diets in general tend to be part fact and part marketing story. The research behind the rationale for carbohydrate-restricted diets is limited at best. The fact is that insulin sends glucose into cells, including fat cells. The marketing hype is that because insulin is mostly secreted when carbohydrates are consumed, the more carbohydrates a person eats, the more glucose will be sent to the fat cells. Therefore, the message conveyed is carbohydrates must make people fat. However, there is no research to verify this claim. The distinction is critical for clinicians to understand if they are going to be able to translate diets and myths for the patient. Thus far, research has shown that excess calories increase body weight, not excess protein, carbohydrates, or fat per se. Likewise, there is little empirical evidence that ketosis, no matter how small, results in reduced hunger. The research on ketosis and hunger is equivocal at best. However, some scientific studies do point to protein as being more satiating than other macronutrients (12–14).

In the case study, if Janice is referring to fad diets that are very low in carbohydrate and very high in fat, then it is important for her to understand the potential risks inherent in those types of diets. For Janice, the risks include the fact that the fats tend to be saturated and could worsen her hyperlipidemia. Also, she would have to be compliant in taking the vitamins, potassium, and extra calcium she would need to supplement what she will be missing in the diet.

Carbohydrate-restricted diets may produce more weight loss than other diets, partly because of the diuresing effect (15). If there are other reasons for a greater effect, they are as yet unknown. However—and herein may be one lesson to be learned—in comparison with the more moderate diets, it may be easier for some people to follow a diet that eliminates a whole category of food. Furthermore, the theoretical cardiac risks of such a diet short-term may be less than researchers once thought (16,17). That fact alone may bode well for the clinician who needs all the tools available to help a patient lose weight and keep it off (see Table 5B.1 for various popular diets and the differences in macronutrients).

Glycemic Diets

Glycemic Index

In the case study above, Janice has confused the issue of low-carbohydrate diets with the glycemic-controlled ones, which is a common problem. Given the current proclivity for eating so many carbohydrates (mostly in the form of low-fiber starch and simple sugar, not in the form of vegetables or whole grains), it is understandable that so many diets suggest limiting them. However, there is a significant difference between diets that limit low-fiber carbohydrates and those that restrict or even eliminate all carbohydrates equally.

The GI diet is a moderate eating plan similar to US Department of Agriculture (USDA) recommendations: high-fiber starch, small portions, lots of vegetables, lean meats, and fish (18,19). But the GI uses a system of ranking all carbohydrate foods with numbers that indicate the degree to which they raise blood sugar immediately after eating them. These numbers are determined by taking the blood sugar responses to different foods eaten by a certain number of individuals and averaging them. The responses are then compared with a reference food: either white bread or glucose. One of the differences in accuracy of the GI may be that different reference foods are used to assess the GI (20).

A food with a low GI (<50) is more desirable than a food with higher numbers, because foods with lower numbers slow the release of glucose into the blood stream, thereby reducing the surges of insulin necessary to remove larger amounts of glucose. Proponents of this type of eating suggest that this flattening of the insulin curve increases satiety, thereby reducing consumption of extra calories. Studies investigating levels of satiety resulting from the consumption of a low-glycemic diet are few, and the number of subjects is small. The results of these studies do suggest that low-glycemic diets lower

Table 5B.1. Macronutrient Distribution for 8 Different 1,600-Calorie Popular Diets*

	Atkins	Zone	Sugar Busters	Ornish	USDA Pyramid	Low-Glycemic	DASH	Volumetrics
Protein (g) (%)	134 (33)	120 (30)	100 (25)	60 (15)	72 (18)	112 (28)	72 (18)	80 (20)
Carbohydrate (g) (%)	35 (9)	160 (40)	140 (35)	290 (80)	236 (59)	230 (58)	208 (52)	240 (60)
Fat (g) (%)	105 (58)	53 (30)	70 (40)	10 (6)	43 (24)	24 (14)	53 (30)	36 (20)
Fiber (g)	8	30	25	40	32	25	30	33

*This chart is an amalgam of many different menus and reports. All data are based on a hypothetical 1,600 calorie/day weight-loss diet.

the insulin response to certain ingested carbohydrates, but the results are inconclusive regarding decreasing hunger and promoting weight loss (21).

Examples of some foods and their GI number are shown in Table 5B.2. An expanded list can be found on http://www.glycemicindex.com.

Glycemic Load

Another concept along the same theme that is gaining recognition is glycemic load (GL). This number is derived from multiplying the GI of a food by the number of grams of available carbohydrate in that food. Whereas the GI requires both the portions of the reference food and test foods to contain the same amount of carbohydrates, thereby inflating the portion of the test food, the GL defines the glycemic effect of a regular serving size of the food. Therefore, the GL is the product of the amount of carbohydrate in a single serving and the GI of that food. Some foods that may have a high GI in actuality have a low GL, because of the small amount of carbohydrate per serving of food. The perfect example of this is the carrot. In order to reach the standard 50 g of carbohydrate to obtain the GI of 95, a person would have to eat 1½ pounds of carrots (22,23). In fact, a single serving of carrots has only 8 available grams of carbohydrate, and therefore has a low GL (23).

There is no evidence to show that diets low in GI or GL are better than others for weight loss, but the types of food suggested are high in fiber and protein and low in saturated fats, which makes them nutritionally balanced diets. However, they can be difficult diets to follow, for both the clinician and the client, for the following reasons: (1) only about 750 different foods have been tested for their GI, omitting thousands of foods; (2) one person's glycemic response to a food may be markedly different from the next person's; (3) combining foods with different glycemic numbers, such as baked potatoes with sour cream, results in a different number from that if eating the food alone; and (4) different values of GI are listed in different publications. The latter problem results from a number of issues: (1) the two dif-

Table 5B.2. Glycemic Index for Selected Foods

Food	Glycemic Index
Carrot	95
Baked potato	93
Spaghetti	41
Chocolate milk	34

ferent reference values; (2) difference in blood samples (capillary vs venous); (3) the brand of food; and (4) the study or studies from which the GI was obtained. Using carrots again, in one study the GI was 92 ± 20, whereas in the newest study it resulted in a GI of 32 ± 5 (23).

Case Study. Janice—Part II: Guiding Principles

The first question to be addressed is what diet does Janice want? Does she want one that eliminates virtually all carbohydrates or one that eliminates high-glycemic foods?

Flexibility

A low-carbohydrate diet can be one that is merely lower than the total amount of carbohydrates the person has been consuming already, or it can be very-low-carbohydrate, as in the Atkins diet. A GI diet is not low in carbohydrates; rather it is high in fibrous carbohydrates and reduces those carbohydrates that are low in fiber. The fact that Janice suggested both a low-carbohydrate and a glycemic diet probably means that she is less aware of the differences and is willing to eat a variety of foods if her high-risk ones are eliminated. That gives the professional a little more room to maneuver.

When asked about her "problem" carbohydrates, Janice admits that vegetables, milk, and fruit are not problem foods for her, and she would be happy to increase them in her new diet. She reports that bread is the worst offender and that she tends to nibble on starchy foods, such as crackers, pretzels, and bagels.

Health Status

Janice is certainly healthy enough to follow a diet for weight loss. However, if she were to follow a carbohydrate-restricted diet, she would need to be monitored more closely by her physician for potential risks of electrolyte loss, dehydration, and hyperuricemia (see Chapter 3: Clinical Monitoring).

Nutritional Completeness

If Janice can eat more fibrous foods, such as vegetables, fruits, and small portions of whole grains, this diet will improve her total nutrition.

The Big Picture

Janice is interested in reducing the risk of diabetes and cardiovascular disease, both of which run in the family; and she wants to reduce her hunger. She wants to do this within the structure of family life and somehow make it realistic enough to maintain her weight loss.

A glycemic diet is probably not appropriate for Janice, because it takes a lot of work to look up every food and to control portions in order to lose weight. Choosing between "bad" and "good" carbohydrates might be tiring for this busy woman, who does not want to think more about food than she already does. However, there is no sense in restricting all carbohydrates if she has expressed a willingness to increase her intake of vegetables and fruit.

Weight Loss

Anything the professional can do to make adherence to a lower-calorie diet easier will help Janice attain weight loss. If eliminating certain foods is the answer, then perhaps Janice can omit all starch at lunch and dinner. This lowers carbohydrates, as Janice has requested, and clarifies food boundaries, similarly to a popular diet. But it also increases the fiber in her diet, which concurs with some of the guidelines for a glycemic diet. Furthermore, both Janice and the provider believe that these changes will actually improve her nutritional picture. The diet itself is not low in carbohydrates, just lower in comparison with Janice's former diet.

Case Study. Janice—Part III: The Standard Dietary Plan With a Low-Carbohydrate Twist

Janice's diet prescription is approximately 1,500 kcal—25% protein, 30% fat, and 45% carbohydrate—which adheres to the guidelines set by the Institute of Medicine's Dietary Reference Intakes (24). The diet consists of three dairy servings, six vegetable servings, three fruit servings, three servings of cereal or beans, two to three meat servings, and five fat servings. To increase the novelty of this diet, the clinician might call it the "no bread diet" and instruct Janice to omit bread products for the next several weeks.

The "No Bread Diet"

This plan would include breakfast, which Janice does not usually eat. For example, for breakfast she would have two servings of high-fiber cereal plus a medium banana and nonfat milk. For lunch, a large salad with 4 oz of grilled chicken, $\frac{1}{3}$ cup garbanzo beans, 1 tablespoon of sesame seeds, and a measured amount of salad dressing. For the midafternoon snack, fat-free yogurt. For dinner, 4 oz of grilled fish, seasoned steamed vegetables, mixed greens and tomato salad. And for the evening snack, a large apple and a glass of nonfat milk.

Case Study. Robert—Part I

Robert is a 50-year-old man who is 70 inches tall and weighs 200 lb. His BMI is 29, indicative of overweight. His most recent lab results show his serum cholesterol is 199 mg/dL; his LDL-C is 121 mg/dL; and his HDL-C is 32 mg/dL. His serum glucose is <100 mg/dL, fasting. His serum triglycerides are 230 mg/dL. His blood pressure is 140/90.

Weight History

Robert has never had to lose weight before, although he has tried to reduce red meat because it seemed like the healthful thing to do. At a recent doctor's visit, he was diagnosed with hypertension and dyslipidemia, and his physician told him to lose 25 pounds or he would need medication for his blood pressure.

Dietary Patterns

Before his diagnosis, Robert's typical intake was coffee and orange juice in the morning and a large, deli-style sandwich with chips and a soft drink for lunch. For dinner, he often bought a meal at an upscale supermarket or went out with friends or clients. He usually had a beer or two after work and an occasional bowl of ice cream at bedtime. On business trips, he ate breakfasts of muffins or sweet rolls and drank more alcohol at night. He says he is now ready to make dramatic changes.

Robert lives alone and is willing to do only minimal food preparation. When he heard that he might have to take a blood pressure pill, he was motivated to make some changes on his own. Robert has been ordering fish more often in restaurants and limiting himself to one beer or cocktail a couple of times per week. He has cut out his chips with lunch and has also tried to eliminate butter but thinks bread and potatoes taste dry without it. He has stopped eating ice cream before bed.

Dietary Request

Robert's colleague from work, who recently had a heart attack, was following the Ornish diet (25) and had already lost 10 pounds. Robert feels highly motivated because he does not want to take hypertensive medications, but he is not sure he can follow such a restrictive diet.

Professional Dilemma

This kind of diet works best for detail-oriented clients with considerable time to shop for and prepare food, but it tends to be difficult for people who travel frequently or do little home food preparation. Although Robert wants to discuss the Ornish diet, it is not at all clear that he understands the full extent to which he would have to reduce fat, salt, and sugar. Therefore, Robert may not be a good match for this kind of diet.

All diets need careful food selection to balance nutrients as well as possible. Fat-restricted diets are no different. These types of diets can be low in calcium, vitamin B-12, zinc, and fat-soluble vitamins, although their emphasis on whole grains, legumes, fruits, and vegetables offers the potential for rich phytochemical intake. Robert would need a lot of nutritional guidance to be able to choose appropriately.

Fat-Restricted Diets

The popularity of diets with 10% fewer calories from fat is waning, but they remain a valid option for some clients, especially those who hope to reduce cardiovascular risk factors as well as weight (26). A recent USDA study (27) demonstrated that participants on very-low-fat, high-carbohydrate diets had a lower BMI and consumed 300 fewer kcal/day than those on very-low-carbohydrate diets.

Critics have suggested that a very-low-fat, high-carbohydrate diet may increase serum triglycerides (28), but in most studies, weight loss of any kind will reduce triglycerides as well as other blood lipids, glucose, and blood pressure (29).

In the above case study, Robert wants to reduce fat and improve his blood pressure. The clinician may want to discuss other options, such as the Dietary Approaches to Stop Hypertension (DASH) diet (30). The DASH diet has been shown to reduce hypertension when compared with a low-sodium, traditional diet or one that emphasizes fruits and vegetables (31). The DASH diet is even richer in vegetables and fruits, but it also emphasizes small portions of whole grains, nuts, and low-fat dairy. Guidelines suggest 8 to 11 servings of fruits and vegetables (30).

Robert wants to hear other alternatives, including the Mediterranean diet, which is high in monounsaturated fats, and Volumetrics (32), developed by Barbara Rolls, PhD (see Table 5B.1). Volumetrics emphasizes foods with a high water content that are also high in fiber, such as fruits, vegetables, low-fat milk, and cooked grains, as well as lean meats, poultry, fish, and beans. By adding bulk and keeping the energy density low, satiety may improve.

Case Study. Robert—Part II: Guiding Principles

Flexibility

It is obvious that Robert does not need to follow the rigidity of a very-low-fat diet in order to lose weight and that this kind of diet would not be practical with his lifestyle. However, this is an opportunity to educate him better about fats and fiber. This can all be done within the context of a lower-fat diet.

Health Status

A lower-fat diet is a good choice for Robert. Although his triglycerides are high, a higher-fiber carbohydrate diet may help to reduce them (33). Furthermore, weight loss will reduce his blood pressure. It is important to ensure that when Robert does eat fat, that most be monounsaturated and fish oils.

Nutritional Completeness

A low-fat diet is not necessarily a low-calorie diet or a nutritionally complete one. Emphasizing portion control, higher-fiber food choices, and vegetables rather than all low-fat foods can help Robert improve the nutritional value of his diet while losing weight.

Big Picture

Robert has already made healthful changes. What are the next steps that he can take while remaining realistic about his lifestyle?

Weight Loss

For Robert, the three biggest issues remain adherence to the structure of the diet while he travels as well as at home, increasing monounsaturated fats while decreasing total calories, and portion control.

Robert agrees that he needs fairly simple guidelines and is not the type to be fastidious about food. He would rather reduce his options than be overly concerned with making the waiter understand his request. He is willing to try any diet, as long as changes can be made quickly if there are no results. He wants to reduce his blood pressure, and he wants to lose weight. His goal is to do both by the time he sees his physician in 6 weeks.

After stepping on the scale, Robert is pleased to discover that the small changes he made before his first visit to the clinician has already produced a weight loss of about 5 lb. Now he is more motivated than ever.

Case Study. Robert—Part III: The Dietary Plan With a Low-Fat Twist

Robert needs clear choices that are easy to find and that require no preparation. For breakfast, he agrees that cereal with fruit and nonfat milk is his best choice. The clinician can suggest several ready-to-eat whole-grain cereals that he could order at hotels. To decrease calories from fat at lunch, he feels he can easily order a turkey sandwich on regular whole-wheat bread with mustard plus a salad or tomato-based soup. Once or twice each week he will have a salad as a main course. For dinner, he will order fish three times per week. He will keep alcohol to no more than two glasses of wine with dinner on weekends.

He agrees to eat a piece of whole fruit or a large serving of vegetables at each meal and to do without bread and butter in a restaurant. Robert will keep individual one-serving bags of nuts and raisins in his briefcase if he gets hungry, as well as a few nutrition bars in case he gets stuck at an airport.

A pact is made with the clinician: if Robert does not lose weight by his next visit, a more stringent regimen will be adopted. This is an important step. All popular diets have "bad foods" that make adherence clear—if the individual steps over the line, then he or she does not get the effects of the diet. In Robert's case, the line may not be clear enough, and there may still be too much choice. If need be, the clinician can make the diet simpler, such as eating only half of everything on the plate or ordering only fish when in a restaurant. As in Janice's case, the clinician is not giving Robert a popular diet per se. Instead, Robert is following a realistic modification of the diet he originally wanted.

Liquid Diets

Although weight loss is a matter of calories consumed vs calories expended, the structure and the form of the diet can improve adherence to reduced-calorie regimens. Two types of diets—very-low-calorie diets (VLCDs) and meal replacements—attempt to improve adherence by confining food choices to preportioned, ready-made products. Both are described later in this chapter as possibilities for Janice and Robert.

Very-Low-Calorie Diets

VLCDs were developed in the 1920s as a way of obtaining larger weight losses than ordinarily seen with regular food diets, but without the complications that might occur with total starvation. VLCDs are defined as < 800 kcal (34) and > 400 kcal (35). Given their low-calorie content, the weight criteria for a VLCD is BMI ≥ 30.

Nutritional Picture. The most frequently used VLCDs are liquid formulas (eg, Optifast, Novartis Nutrition Corp, Minneapolis, MN 55440; HMR, Health Management Resources, Boston MA, 02111). The liquid VLCDs have the advantage of containing more complete nutrition than prepackaged bars or meals. Unlike regular food, where the bitterness of additional nutrients can adversely affect taste, blenderized liquids can be made to be palatable, even with the addition of more macronutrients and micronutrients. They are usually in powder form, mixed with water, and consumed four to six times daily. They serve as the sole source of nutrition.

These formulas provide approximately 14 to 18 g of good-quality protein per packet, or 70 to 90 g/day, usually from milk, soy, and egg sources. Liquid VLCDs contain at least enough carbohydrate to avoid ketosis and are usually 50% to 60% carbohydrate. Carbohydrates tend to be in the form of maltodextrins, as well as sucrose and either saccharine and/or aspartame, and usually contain little or no fiber. Liquid VLCDS also contain enough essential fatty acids to meet requirements and provide more than 100% of the recommended dietary allowances (RDAs) for vitamins and minerals. A one-a-day multivitamin can be prescribed as a safety precaution, but any other supplements should be evaluated and possibly discontinued to avoid excessive doses, particularly of calcium.

Re-entry to Regular Food. VLCDs are usually prescribed for 12 to 16 weeks, at which point a re-entry diet of part formula, part food is prescribed until the patient is weaned off all formula. The goal is to slowly reintroduce enough regular food to equal 1,200 to 1,500 kcal/day. Refeeding generally takes 4 to 6 weeks but depends on the patient. Calories are increased by 100 to 150 kcal/day. For example, in the first week, the patient might reduce one packet of formula per day, replacing it with 2 to 3 oz of white-meat chicken and ½ cup of steamed vegetables. Or, total calories may need to be increased by adding food to formula packets. For example, a banana may be added to a formula, or a small meal of protein and vegetables may be prescribed in addition to formula calories. Eventually, as the stomach adapts to regular food, salads and other raw vegetables, as well as seasonings, are reintroduced.

Anyone starting any diet for weight loss should see a physician, but diets with less than 1,000 kcal/day should include frequent physician supervision during weight loss, to avoid the greater risks inherent with VLCDs, such as hypokalemia, cardiac arrhythmia, and lean tissue loss (see Chapter 3: Clinical Monitoring).

Short-term Weight Losses. VLCDs are effective in inducing larger short-term weight losses (36). VLCDs result in weight losses of 13 to 23 kg, as compared with the 9 to 13 kg losses of low-calorie diets (1,000 to 1,500 kcal).

Long-term Weight Losses. There is some debate about the outcome of long-term maintenance of weight loss after VLCDs. Most earlier research has shown complete or higher weight regain. However, in recent reviews, weight-loss maintenance after VLCDs differs considerably, depending on intensity of follow-up (37–41). More studies need to be done to compare the efficacy of weight-loss maintenance to length of time on VLCDs and the use of meal replacements and pharmacotherapy to help maintain the larger weight losses.

Liquid Meal Replacements

A liquid formula can also be substituted for one or two meals, with the directions to eat a "sensible meal" for either lunch or dinner. Meal replacements can be found over-the-counter, in drugstores and supermarkets. Low-calorie diets can be defined as providing 800 to 1,500 kcal/day. Like VLCDs, there are many incarnations of these meal replacements, from liquid to powder to bars to prepackaged frozen and freeze-dried meals. The usual meal replacement now includes 0 to 5 g fiber, 10 to 14 g protein (microwavable meals may have more), 25% to 30% of RDAs for vitamins and minerals, and the rest carbohydrate. Although there are a few formulas that are higher in fat, most contain less than 5 g fat and are high in sugar. These formulas are usually milk-based and high in calcium. On average, they range from 150 to 250 kcal.

Short-term Weight Losses. Meal replacements, when used appropriately, can be very successful. In one study that compared weight loss using free packaged foods vs giving money per visit, packaged foods proved to be the more successful (42). In studies comparing the use of SlimFast with traditional low-calorie diets, the SlimFast groups showed significantly better weight loss (43).

Long-term Weight Losses. The data on meal replacement for one meal per day show good weight maintenance compared with those who attempt weight-loss maintenance without a meal replacement. One study compared the efficacy of SlimFast with the efficacy of traditional food diets prescribed in either a physician's office or a dietitian's support group, and found that the use of one or two meal replacements daily promoted significantly improved weight loss and maintenance (44). Other studies looking at long-term weight-loss efficacy using meal replacements have shown significant success for up to 5 years (45,46).

Case Study. Robert and Janice—Final Thoughts

Although Janice fits the VLCD criteria for weight and Robert does not, Janice is not interested in a VLCD. She wants to eat a meal with her family, and she does not want to take time out to see the physician and get the necessary follow-up blood tests that are required as part of good supervision on a VLCD.

However, Janice thinks that a meal replacement for breakfast and lunch might work. First, she would be eating something nutritious for breakfast; second, a meal replacement for lunch would be an easy and inexpensive choice. An over-the-counter formula would help Janice increase her calcium consumption, and, if she adds a fruit with her formula, she will increase her fiber as well as her vitamin intake.

For Robert, a meal replacement can be used periodically on business trips when he arrives at his hotel late at night, when he is stuck in the airport during a delay, or when he does not have time for lunch between business meetings. Robert elects to use formula bars as meal replacements because these are easier for him to carry in his travel bag.

At approximately 6 months, it is common for weight to plateau. (The literature is clear: no matter what the study, how intense the behavioral or nutrition involvement, a plateau is common and usual.) Whether these plateaus are physical or psychological is unknown, but their occurrence is virtually guaranteed. Therefore, it is helpful to discuss plateaus with clients before they occur.

Suppose Robert has lost 20 pounds following a low-fat diet, but for 2 months now his weight has not changed and he is getting frustrated. He reports to the clinician that he is still following the same dietary regimen and he does not understand why he is not losing more weight. Robert's immediate reaction is to push himself to lose more weight, but he is already feeling deprived. The clinician thinks that Robert should accept maintenance as a success and continue to maintain until he is truly ready to work at further weight loss. After all, if Robert wants to lose more weight, he should return to making more accurate food records, measuring portions, and exercising more frequently.

It is helpful to think about a new routine at times of plateau. Even if Robert cannot lose any more weight, he will still have to be ready to battle to maintain his weight loss. For example, this is where a meal replacement can be useful. Not only does it limit calories, but it helps to focus the client, clarifying food boundaries that have become amorphous. Other possibilities might be a lower-carbohydrate diet in Robert's case, or a higher-carbohydrate diet in Janice's case.

Whatever happens, it is important to remind the client that a plateau means that the diet did its job: in Robert's case, he has lost 10% of his weight and his blood pressure is within normal limits without medication. As partners, Robert and his clinician have met the guiding principles—and Robert is healthier for having done so.

Final Note

As long as the majority of Americans remain obese, discussions about the best diet will abound. In reality, weight loss is simply a juggling of the calories contained in fats, proteins, and carbohydrates—calories in vs calories out. Whether one macronutrient confers better health than another is being hotly debated. Regardless, a clinician must be prepared to hear the wanton cry: "Help me with the newest popular diet!" If clinicians are not prepared to be flexible, they take the risk of losing more than a client; they lose the opportunity to guide someone to better health.

References

1. Freedman MR, King J, Kennedy E. Popular diets: a scientific review. *Obes Res*. 2001;9(Suppl 1):1S–40S.
2. National Institutes of Health, National Heart, Lung, and Blood Institute. *Clinical Guidelines on the Identification, Evaluation, and Treatment of Overweight and Obesity in Adults*. Bethesda, Md: National Institutes of Health; 2002. NIH Publication No. 00-4084
3. Knowler WC, Barrett-Conner E, Fowler SE, Hamman RF, Lachin JM, Walker EA, Nathan DM. Reduction in the incidence of type 2 diabetes with lifestyle intervention or metformin. *New Engl J Med*. 2002;346:393–403.
4. Wadden TA, Letizia KA . Predictors of attrition and weight loss in patients treated by moderate and severe caloric restriction. In: Wadden TA, Van Itallie TB, eds. *Treatment of the Seriously Obese Patient*. New York, NY: Guilford Press; 1992:383–410.
5. Cummings S, Parham ES, Strain GW. Position of the American Dietetic Association: weight management. *J Am Diet Assoc*. 2002;108:1145–1155.
6. Aronne LJ. Classification of obesity and assessment of obesity-related health risks. *Obes Res*. 2002;10 (suppl 2):105S–115S.
7. Reaven G. Metabolic syndrome: pathophysiology and implications for management of cardiovascular disease. *Circulation*. 2002;106:286–288.
8. Atkins RC. *Dr. Atkins New Diet Revolution*. New York, NY: Avon Books; 1992.
9. Brand-Miller J, Wolever TMS, Calgiuri S, Foster-Powell K. *The Glucose Revolution*. New York, NY: Marlowe & Co; 1996.
10. Bravata DM, Sanders L, Huang J, Krumholz HM, Olkin I, Gardner CD, Bravata DM. Efficacy and safety of low-carbohydrate diets: a systematic review. *JAMA*. 2003;289:1837–1850.
11. Van Itallie TB, Nufert TH. Ketones: metabolism's "ugly duckling." *Nutr Rev*. 2003 (in press).
12. Long SJ, Jeffcoat AR, Millward DJ. Effect of habitual dietary-protein intake on appetite and satiety. *Appetite*. 2000;35:79–88.
13. Latner JD, Schwartz M. The effects of a high-carbohydrate, high-protein or balanced lunch upon later food intake and hunger rating, *Appetite*. 1999;33: 119–128.

14. Lang V, Bellisle F, Oppert JM, Craplet C, Bornet FR, Slama G, Guy-Grand B. Satiating effect of proteins in healthy subjects: a comparison of egg albumin, casein, gelatin, soy protein, pea protein, wheat gluten. *Am J Clin Nutr*. 1998; 67:1197–1204.

15. Van Itallie TB, Yang MU. Diet and weight loss. *N Engl J Med*. 1977;297: 1158–1161.

16. Foster GD, Wyatt HR, Hill JO, McGuckin BG, Brill C, Mohammed BS, Szapary PO, Rader DJ, Edman JS, Klein S. A randomized trial of a low-carbohydrate diet for obesity. *N Engl J Med*. 2003;348:2082–2090.

17. Samaha FF, Iqbal N, Seshadri P, Chicano KL, Daily DA, McGrory J, Williams T, Williams M, Gracely EJ, Stern L. A low-carbohydrate as compared with a low-fat diet in severe obesity. *N Engl J Med*. 2003;348:2074–2081.

18. Ludwig DS. Dietary glycemic index and obesity. *J Nutr*. 2000;130(2S Suppl): 280S–283S.

19. Agus MSD, Swain JF, Larson CL, Eckert EA, Ludwig DS. Dietary composition and physiologic adaptations to energy restriction. *Am J Clin Nutr*. 2000;71: 901–907.

20. Pi-Sunyer FX. Glycemic index and disease. *Am J Clin Nutr*. 2002;76:290S–298S.

21. Brand-Miller JC, Holt SH, Pawlak DB, McMillan J. Glycemic index and obesity. *Am J Clin Nutr*. 2002;76:281S–285S.

22. Jane E. Brody. Personal health: fear not that carrot, potato, or ear of corn. *New York Times*. June 11, 2002.

23. Foster-Powell K, Holt SHA, Brand-Miller JC. International table of glycemic index and glycemic load values: 2002. *Am J Clin Nutr*. 2002;76:5–56.

24. Institute of Medicine, National Academy of Sciences. *Dietary Reference Intakes for Energy, Carbohydrate, Fiber, Fat, Fatty Acids, Cholesterol, Protein, and Amino Acids* (prepublication version). Washington, DC: National Academies Press; 2002.

25. Ornish D. *Dr. Dean Ornish's Program for Reversing Heart Disease*. New York, NY: Ballantine Books; 1990.

26. Ornish D, Scherwitz LW, Billings JH, Brown SE, Gould KL, Merritt TA, Sparler S, Armstrong WT, Ports TA, Kirkeeide RL, Hogeboom C, Brand RJ. Intensive lifestyle changes for reversal of coronary heart disease. *JAMA*. 1998;280: 2001–2007.

27. Bowman SA, Spence JT. A comparison of low-carbohydrate vs. high-carbohydrate diets: energy restriction, nutrient quality and correlation to body mass index. *J Am Coll Nutr*. 2002;21:268–274.

28. McLaughlin T, Abbrasi F, Lamenola C, Yeni-Komshian H, Reaven G. Carbohydrate-induced hypertriglyceridemia: an insight into the link between plasma insulin and triglyceride concentrations. *J Clin Endocrinol Metab*. 2000;85: 3085–3088.

29. Bonow RO, Eckel RH. Diet, obesity, and cardiovascular disease. *N Engl J Med*. 2003;348:2057–2058.

30. Lin PH, Aickin M, Champagne C, Craddick S, Sacks FM, McCarron P, Most-Windhauser MM, Rukenbrod F, Haworth L; DASH-Sodium Collaborative Re-

search Group. Food group sources of nutrients in the dietary patterns of the DASH-Sodium trial. *J Am Diet Assoc.* 2003;103:488–496.

31. Appel LJ, Champagne CM, Harsha DW, Cooper LS, Obarzanek E, Elmer PJ, Stevens VJ, Vollmer WM, Lin PH, Svetkey LP, Stedman SW, Young DR. Effects of comprehensive lifestyle modification on blood pressure control: main results of the PREMIER clinical trial. *JAMA.* 2003;289:2083–2093.

32. Rolls B, Barnett RA. *The Volumetrics: Weight-Control Plan.* New York, NY: HarperCollins Publishers; 2000.

33. Anderson JW. Dietary fiber prevents carbohydrate-induced hypertriglyceridemia. *Curr Atheroscler Rep.* 2000;2:536–541.

34. National Task Force on the Prevention and Treatment of Obesity. Very-low-calorie diets. *JAMA.* 1993;270:967–974.

35. Kushner R. Very-low-calorie diets. In: Bessesen DH, Kushner R, eds. *Evaluation and Management of Obesity.* Philadelphia, Pa: Hanley & Belfus; 2002: 71–72.

36. Wadden TA, Brownell KD, Foster GD. Obesity: responding to the global epidemic. *J Consult Clin Psychol.* 2002;70:510–525.

37. Saris WH. Very-low-calorie diets and sustained weight loss. *Obes Res.* 2001;9(Suppl 4):295S–301S.

38. Pekkarinen T, Mustajoki P. Comparison of behavior therapy with and without very-low-energy diet in the treatment of morbid obesity. A 5-year outcome. *Arch Intern Med.* 1997;157:1581–1585.

39. Mustajoki P, Pekkarine T. Very-low-energy diets in the treatment of obesity. *Obes Rev.* 2001;2:61–72.

40. Ayyad C, Anderson T. Long-term efficacy of dietary treatment of obesity: a systematic review of studies published between 1931 and 1999. *Obes Rev.* 2000;1:261–272.

41. Finer N. Low-calorie diets and sustained weight loss. *Obes Res.* 2001; 9(Suppl 4):290S–294S.

42. Jeffrey RW, Wing RR. Long-term effects of interventions for weight loss using food provision and monetary incentives. *J Consult Clin Psychol.* 1995;63: 793–796.

43. Rothacker DQ, Staniszewski BA, Ellis PK. Liquid meal replacement vs traditional model for women who cannot maintain eating habit changes. *J Am Diet Assoc.* 2001;101:345–347.

44. Ashley JM, St. Jeor ST, Perumean-Chaney SP, Schrage J, Bovee V. Meal replacements in weight intervention. *Obes Res.* 2001;9:312S–320S.

45. Rothacker DQ. Five-year self-management of weight using meal replacements: comparison with matched controls in rural Wisconsin. *Nutrition.* 2000;16:344–348.

46. Fletchner-Mors M, Ditschuneit HH, Johnson TD, Suchard MA, Adler G. Metabolic and weight-loss effects of long-term dietary intervention in obese patients: four-year results. *Obes Res.* 2000;8:399–402.

Chapter 6
Physical Activity

PART A. Overview

Steven N. Blair, PED

Physical Activity and Health

It is no surprise that regular physical activity is a cornerstone of good health and function. Human beings have existed for at least 2 million years. Human evolution in the grassy savannahs of the temperate zone, and selection pressures led to the development of a genus that is ideally designed for a hunter-gatherer lifestyle. It is only within about the past 10,000 years that humans began to develop agriculture, congregate in larger settlements, and ultimately form complex societies. The period of the industrial revolution began about 250 years ago and led, in turn, to mass production, urbanization, the internal combustion engine, and the computer and telecommunications revolution of the past 25 years. Although civilization has brought many advantages, humans are simply not animals designed to live in an environment with the hectic pace of modern life, abundant and cheap food, and low requirements for energy expenditure to sustain life.

There is now conclusive evidence that a sedentary and unfit way of life increases the risk of developing numerous chronic diseases (coronary heart disease, stroke, hypertension, colon cancer, type 2 diabetes), decreases longevity, interferes with body weight regulation, and leads to a loss of physical function and independence in the later years of life (1–3). The strong, independent, graded, biologically plausible risks associated with low levels of physical activity and fitness, accompanied by the high prevalence of the sedentary lifestyle in modern societies, leads to high population attributable risk for inactivity. Thus, a sedentary and unfit lifestyle is one of the major public health problems of the 21st century.

Physical Activity and Weight Management

Regulation of body weight is dependent on maintaining energy balance. The laws of thermodynamics dictate that if energy intake is greater than energy expenditure, the excess energy must be stored. Excess energy is stored as adipose tissue, and we have a large capacity to store energy. Each kilogram of adipose tissue will yield about 7,700 kcal when metabolized, or about three to four times the average daily energy requirement of adults. The energy intake side of the energy balance equation is based on the caloric value of ingested food.

On the expenditure side of the equation, total energy expenditure (TEE) is determined by the resting metabolic rate (resting energy expenditure, or REE), the thermic effect of food (the energy cost of digesting and processing food), and the amount of physical activity (activity energy expenditure, or AEE). AEE takes many forms. It can arise from the minimal muscular movement required for tasks of daily living, such as grooming, dressing, feeding, and basic household chores. Earning a living, being a caretaker, or other routine requirements of life add to AEE, as do recreation, sports, and other leisure-time pursuits.

In modern societies, the greatest contribution to overall energy expenditure is from REE, and energy expenditure from AEE often is low. Although REE is relatively immutable, AEE can be increased greatly. It seems clear that requirements for AEE declined steadily during the 20th century. It is quite likely that this trend accelerated toward the end of the century, because of the increasing use of labor-saving devices at home and at work, along with increasingly inactive leisure-time activities (4). This trend of declining AEE, and consequently declining TEE, especially in the presence of a ubiquitous food environment, has led to many individuals being in chronic, positive energy balance. The result has been increases in the prevalence of overweight and obesity. Furthermore, it is also probable that average TEE levels have dropped so low that appetite regulation to match intake with expenditure becomes difficult, if not nearly impossible, for an increasing numbers of individuals. Therefore, any strategy to improve weight management must include substantial emphasis on increasing AEE, and this applies to the primary prevention of weight gain, to weight-loss efforts, to maintenance of weight loss, and to enhancing health for individuals of all sizes and shapes.

Physical Activity in Primary Prevention

It is logical to assume that sedentary lifestyles contribute to a positive energy balance and are an important cause of the increasing numbers of overweight individuals. Unfortunately, data to clearly specify the causes of weight gain are sparse and often inconsistent (this applies to both sides of the energy balance equation) (4). The lack of data is likely a result of the difficulty of measuring energy intake and energy expenditure in large representative populations or even in sizable clinical samples. The error of measurement for both diet and physical activity is large, and a small daily positive energy balance that is undetectable by current methodology can still result in substantial weight gain over time. For example, a positive daily energy balance of 100 kcal is very difficult to detect, yet would result in a gain of 1 kg (2.2 lb) in about 2.5 months or nearly 5 kg per year. Nonetheless, it seems reasonable to assume that efforts to increase AEE in the population would be a good strategy for the primary prevention of weight gain, and this assumption is supported by studies (5–7).

Physical Activity in Weight-Loss Programs

Most current weight-loss programs place at least some emphasis on increasing physical activity. This is appropriate, although increasing AEE is not especially effective in promoting significant weight loss, at least in the short term. However, physical activity alone or when added to caloric restriction appears to produce about 1 to 2 kg of weight loss during several months, in controlled studies (8). A major reason for which physical activity is relatively ineffective, at least compared with caloric restriction, in short-term weight-loss interventions, is that many overweight or obese individuals are quite sedentary and unfit. This means that they just do not have a large enough "metabolic engine" to burn a large number of calories. For example, it is not uncommon to see obese individuals who have a maximal aerobic power in the range of 5 to 6 multiples of resting metabolic rate (METs). One MET is REE (ie, 3.5 mL $O_2 \times kg^{-1} \times min^{-1}$). Therefore, 5 METs is energy expenditure five times higher than resting metabolism.

Sedentary individuals cannot exercise for more than a few minutes at rates beyond 40% to 50% of their maximal capacity. Therefore, a person with a 5-MET maximal capacity can exercise only at a rate of 2 to 2.5 METs. On average, persons expend 1 kcal/kg of body weight per hour. Thus, if a person weighs 100 kg (220 lb) they will burn only 200 kcal per hour if they walk at 2 mph and about 250 kcal if they walk at 2.5 mph. Walking faster or longer may not be possible for such individuals. In this example, a person would have to walk about 35 hours to metabolize 1 kg (2.2 lb) of body fat. It is critical to note, however, that walking at even 2 mph is better than sitting, which will expend only about 100 kcal per hour for this person.

These facts should not discourage clinicians from recommending physical activity to weight-loss clients. Rather, it is important to set realistic expectations for the effect of exercise. Exercise during weight loss has important benefits. It will likely make participants feel better, and it helps to improve fitness and health. As weight decreases and fitness increases, the metabolic engine will be able to sustain physical activity at a higher-intensity level and for a longer period. This will result in an increased ability to expend calories, so that more fit persons may be able to expend 400 to 500 kcal per hour (9).

There are other important contributions of physical activity in weight-loss programs. Perhaps most importantly, studies show that exercise appears to preferentially mobilize fat from visceral adipose tissue (9,10). Because visceral fat is presumed to be a strong determinant of risk for coronary heart disease (CHD) and diabetes, a small loss of visceral fat may have important health effects. Secondly, regular physical activity during a weight-loss regimen appears to preserve lean body mass and causes more of the weight loss to be from the adipose tissue compartment than from lean body mass (9,10).

Physical Activity in Weight-Loss Maintenance

Regular physical activity makes important contributions to maintaining weight loss after it occurs. Although there are few data from randomized clinical trials on this issue, several lines of evidence strongly indicate that most individuals who have long-term success in maintaining weight loss are highly active. Some impressive data on this point come from doubly labeled water studies of formerly obese persons who have sustained substantial weight losses for an extended period. Doubly labeled water is a precise technique for measuring energy expenditure over a 1- to 2-week period. Studies in the formerly obese indicate that they engage in 60 to 80 minutes of moderate to vigorous physical activity each day (11,12).

The doubly labeled water studies are complemented by data from Hill and Wing, in the National Weight Control Registry (13–15). Individuals in the Registry have lost at least 13.6 kg and have kept it off for at least 1 year. A recent report from the Registry shows that the average weight loss in this group is about 30 kg, and this has been maintained for more than 5 years (16). Thus, the Registry participants have been highly successful in losing weight and in maintaining the loss for an extended time. The characteristics of Registry participants indicate that most of them follow a restricted-calorie diet and are regularly physically active. On average, the participants report expending nearly 3,000 kcal per week in moderate to vigorous physical activity. This amount of activity is likely to require 80 to 90 minutes per day of brisk walking.

Current Public Health Recommendations for Physical Activity

Controlled exercise training studies began in the 1950s. Over the next couple of decades, sufficient data had accumulated to allow quantification and specification of exercise advice. In 1975, the American College of Sports

---

Box 6A.1. Activity, Fitness, and Health at All Levels of BMI: A Researcher's Perspective

The Cooper Institute published several reports during the past 7 years on the importance of physical activity and fitness for individuals in all BMI groups. The first paper on this topic (1995) reported that obese men who were physically fit had a much lower death rate during follow-up than normal-weight men who were unfit (17). Continued investigations show that the results have been remarkably consistent, with the health benefits of activity or fitness extending to individuals in all BMI groups (18,19).

Our most comprehensive report on this topic was a prospective study of 21,925 men examined at the Cooper Clinic and followed for an average of 8 years for mortality, during which time 428 men died (18). Atypical features of this study are that (1) cardiorespiratory fitness was measured by a maximal exercise test on a treadmill; (2) body composition was determined by underwater weighing, the sum of seven skinfolds, or both; and (3) fat distribution was indicated by waist circumference in a subgroup. The primary study results are shown in Figure 6A.1.

The results of our research on the interrelationships between body habitus and cardiorespiratory fitness are consistent with those shown in Figure 6A.1. Within fatness or BMI categories, higher death rates are seen for those who are unfit than for the fit participants. This overall finding persists after adjustment for several potentially confounding factors, after restricting analyses to nonsmokers, and in both women and men (20,21). Most of the obese individuals in our studies are in class I obesity, and we do not know if the findings would apply to those in class II or class III obesity. The conclusion from this research is that a fit and active way of life protects against mortality for individuals who are of normal weight, who are overweight, or who are obese. The clinical message for weight management clients is that regular physical activity may not make you as thin as a model, but it will give you better health.

(Box *continues*)

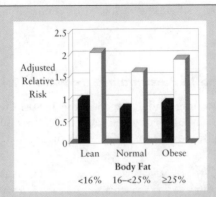

Figure 6A.1. Adjusted relative risks for all-cause mortality for fit and unfit men in categories of percent body fat. Relative risks for the fit men are represented by the black bars and for the unfit men by the white bars. The relative risks are adjusted for age, examination year, smoking status, alcohol intake, and family history of cardiovascular disease.

Adapted with permission from Lee CD, Blair SN, Jackson AS. Cardiorespiratory fitness, body composition, and all-cause and cardiovascular disease mortality in men. *Am J Clin Nutr.* 1999;69:373–380.

Medicine (ACSM) published the first edition of a book on guidelines for exercise prescription (22), followed, in 1978, by a detailed and highly referenced position stand on exercise prescription (23). These two reports have been updated several times by the ACSM, most recently with the 6th edition of the guidelines book in 2000 (24) and the position stand in 1998 (25). The exercise prescription approach to making exercise recommendations is based on sound science, and, if followed, results in physiological adaptations and health benefits. The exercise prescription is based on specifying the frequency, intensity, and duration of exercise. The recommended frequency has changed little over the years, with the general recommended frequency of 3 to 5 days per week. Recommendations for the duration of each session generally have been 20 to 40 minutes. The recommendation for exercise intensity has changed over the years, from about 70% of maximal aerobic power initially to 40% to 50% in the more recent reports. A misinterpretation regarding the exercise prescription approach has been in assuming that the traditional structured quantification of exercise is the only valid way to present exercise recommendations.

Research in the 1990s and a reevaluation of earlier studies led to new public health recommendations for physical activity. The first of these was a report of a workshop organized by the ACSM and the Centers for Disease Control and Prevention (CDC) (2). This report recognized the value of moderate amounts and intensities of physical activity and the usefulness of lifestyle activity in meeting appropriate exercise targets. The public health recommendation for physical activity is that "sedentary adults should accumulate at least 30 minutes of moderate intensity physical activity over the course of most, preferably all, days of the week." Similar recommendations soon followed from the US Surgeon General, the National Institutes of Health, and the American Heart Association (1,3,26).

Important characteristics of the new physical activity recommendations from the ACSM/CDC are that physical activity does not need to be completed all in one session but can be accumulated in sessions of 8 to 10 minutes throughout the day. Furthermore, moderate-intensity activity, such as walking at a pace of 15 to 20 minutes per mile, can provide important health and functional benefits (2,27). Thus, three 10-minute walks provide essentially the same health benefits as one 30-minute walk (2,27). This approach provides an individual with a more flexible way to obtain a healthful dose of exercise. A 10-minute walk to the bus stop, a 10-minute walk to lunch, and a 10-minute walk with a friend or family member after dinner meet the recommendation. Physical activity can be integrated into routine daily activities and does not require the large block of time necessary to get to a fitness center, change, exercise, shower and change, and return to home or work.

It is now clear that intervention methods designed to help individuals develop the cognitive and behavioral skills to integrate more activity into their lives are efficacious in increasing physical activity and fitness and have other beneficial health effects (28,29). Additional research has confirmed the validity of the accumulation recommendation (27). The consensus public health recommendation for physical activity provides a great deal of flexibility in designing and implementing a program to achieve healthful levels of activity. Individuals and health professionals alike can benefit from these new strategies and approaches.

Adapting Physical Activity Recommendations to Weight Management

The question can be posed, Are the ACSM/CDC physical activity recommendations applicable to weight management programs, and if so, how can they be applied? Some clinicians and investigators in the obesity field have criticized the consensus physical activity recommendations because they believe that 30 minutes of moderate-intensity physical activity will not be sufficient to prevent unhealthful weight gain. The Institute of Medicine (IOM) report on dietary reference intakes recommends at least 60 minutes each day of moderately intense physical activity, such as walking/jogging at 4 to 5 mph (30). This amount of physical activity, according to the report, is necessary to prevent weight gain and to achieve the full health benefits of activity. It seems that current data on the issue of how much physical activity is required to prevent unhealthful weight gain are inadequate to resolve this question. (The IOM report also failed to acknowledge adequately the important health benefits that accrue from 30 minutes of moderate-intensity physical activity on most days.)

There are few studies documenting how much activity is required to prevent unhealthful weight gain, but there clearly must be substantial individual variation. Most people can think of someone who has never exercised consistently, has a sedentary job, generally leads a very inactive existence, and yet has not gained any weight over the years or decades. Therefore, some individuals—although probably a small percentage—can maintain their weight with no exercise. Others may exercise 45 to 60 minutes a day and still gain weight with the advancing years. There is no compelling evidence on how much activity is required to maintain a healthy weight throughout life. This question was the topic of a workshop organized by the International Association for the Study of Obesity, and the preliminary report indicates that, although 30 minutes per day may be sufficient for some, a large number of individuals may require 45 to 60 minutes, and some people will require even more (31). Maintaining weight is a good way to monitor whether the physical activity level is sufficient to prevent weight gain. If it is increasing, then one must either increase the activity level or reduce caloric intake.

Maintaining large weight losses in formerly obese individuals likely requires a substantial amount of physical activity. Data from both doubly labeled water studies and from the National Weight Control Registry suggest that 80 to 90 minutes of moderate-intensity exercise per day is necessary in the formerly obese. This is a large time commitment, but it is possible. As individuals exercise regularly and improve their aerobic power, they will be able to expend calories at a higher rate per minute, and the overall exercise time can be reduced.

The most important message for clients is that some exercise is better than none, and more is better than less—up to a point. Overweight or obese individuals who are able to accumulate 30 minutes of moderate-intensity physical activity into their daily routines are not likely to become thin, at least in the short term, in the absence of stringent restriction of caloric intake. However, these individuals should be reminded that the 30 minutes per day is making important contributions to their health.

References

1. NIH Consensus Development Panel on Physical Activity and Cardiovascular Health. Physical activity and cardiovascular health. *JAMA.* 1996;276:241–246.
2. Pate RR, Pratt M, Blair SN, Haskell WL, Macera CA, Bouchard C, Buchner D, Ettinger W, Heath GW, King AC, et al. Physical activity and public health: a recommendation from the Centers for Disease Control and Prevention and the American College of Sports Medicine. *JAMA.* 1995;273:402–407.
3. US Department of Health and Human Services. *Physical Activity and Health: A Report of the Surgeon General,* Atlanta, Ga: US Department of Health and Human Services, Centers for Disease Control and Prevention, National Center for Chronic Disease Prevention and Health Promotion, President's Council on Physical Fitness and Sports; 1996.
4. Blair SN, Nichaman MZ. The public health problem of increasing prevalence rates of obesity and what should be done about it. *Mayo Clin Proc.* 2002;77:109–113.
5. DiPietro L. Physical activity in the prevention of obesity: current evidence and research issues. *Med Sci Sports Exerc.* 1999;31(11 Suppl):S542–S546.
6. DiPietro L, Kohl HW 3rd, Barlow CE, Blair SN. Improvements in cardiorespiratory fitness attenuate age-related weight gain in healthy men and women: the Aerobics Center Longitudinal Study. *Int J Obes Relat Metab Disord.* 1998;22:55–62.
7. Jebb SA, Moore MS. Contribution of a sedentary lifestyle and inactivity to the etiology of overweight and obesity: current evidence and research issues. *Med Sci Sports Exerc.* 1999;31(11 Suppl):S534–S541.
8. Wing RR. Physical activity in the treatment of the adulthood overweight and obesity: current evidence and research issues. *Med Sci Sports Exerc.* 1999; 31(11 Suppl):S547–S552.
9. Ross R, Dagnone D, Jones PJ, Smith H, Paddags A, Hundson R, Janssen I. Reduction in obesity and related comorbid conditions after diet-induced weight loss or exercise-induced weight loss in men. A randomized, controlled trial. *Ann Intern Med.* 2000;133:92–103.
10. Ross R, Janssen I. Is abdominal fat preferentially reduced in response to exercise-induced weight loss? *Med Sci Sports Exerc.* 1999;31(11 Suppl):S568–S572.
11. Schoeller DA. Recent advances from application of doubly labeled water to measurement of human energy expenditure. *J Nutr.* 1999;129:1765–1768.
12. Schoeller DA, Shay K, Kushner RF. How much physical activity is needed to minimize weight gain in previously obese women? *Am J Clin Nutr.* 1997;66:551–556.
13. Klem ML, Wing RR, McGuire MT, Seagle HM, Hill JO. A descriptive study of individuals successful at long-term maintenance of substantial weight loss. *Am J Clin Nutr.* 1997;66:239–246.
14. McGuire MT, Wing RR, Klem ML, Hill JO. Behavioral strategies of individuals who have maintained long-term weight losses. *Obes Res.* 1999;7:334–341.

15. McGuire MT, Wing RR, Klem ML, Seagle HM, Hill JO. Long-term maintenance of weight loss: do people who lose weight through various weight loss methods use different behaviors to maintain their weight? *Int J Obes Relat Metab Disord.* 1998;22:572–577.

16. Wing RR, Hill JO. Successful weight loss maintenance. *Ann Rev Nutr.* 2001; 21:323–342.

17. Barlow CE, Kohl HW 3rd, Gibbons LW, Blair SN. Physical fitness, mortality and obesity. *Int J Obes Relat Metab Disord.* 1995;19(Suppl 4):S41–S44.

18. Lee CD, Blair SN, Jackson AS. Cardiorespiratory fitness, body composition, and all-cause and cardiovascular disease mortality in men. *Am J Clin Nutr.* 1999;69:373–380.

19. Lee CD, Jackson AS, Blair SN. US weight guidelines: is it also important to consider cardiorespiratory fitness? *Int J Obes Relat Metab Disord.* 1998; 22(Suppl 2):S2–S7.

20. Farrell SW, Braun L, Barlow CE, Cheng YJ, Blair SN. The relation of body mass index, cardio fitness, and all-cause mortality in women. *Obes Res.* 2002;10:417–423.

21. Stevens J, Cai J, Evenson KR, Thomas R. Fitness and fatness as predictors of mortality from all causes and from cardiovascular diseases in men and women in the lipid research clinics study. *Am J Epidemiol.* 2002;156: 832–841.

22. American College of Sports Medicine. *Guidelines for Graded Exercise Testing and Exercise Prescription.* Philadelphia, Pa: Lea & Febiger; 1975.

23. American College of Sports Medicine. Position statement on the recommended quantity and quality of exercise for developing and maintaining fitness in healthy adults. *Med Sci Sports.* 1978;10:vii–x.

24. Franklin BA, Whaley MH, Howley ET, eds. American College of Sports Medicine. *ACSM's Guidelines for Exercise Testing and Prescription.* 6th ed. Philadelphia, Pa: Lippincott Williams & Wilkins; 2000.

25. American College of Sports Medicine Position Stand. Exercise and physical activity for older adults. *Med Sci Sports Exerc.* 1998;30:992–1008.

26. Fletcher GF, Balady G, Blair SN, Blumenthal J, Caspersen C, Chaitman B, Epstein S, Sivarajan Froelicher ES, Froelicher VF, Pina IL, Pollack ML. Statement on exercise: benefits and recommendations for physical activity programs for all Americans. A statement for health professionals by the Committee on Exercise and Cardiac Rehabilitation of the Council on Clinical Cardiology, American Heart Association. *Circulation.* 1996;94:857–862.

27. Asikainen TM, Miilunpalo S, Oja P, Rinne M, Pasanen M, Vuori I. Walking trials in postmenopausal women: effect of one vs two daily bouts on aerobic fitness. *Scand J Med Sci Sports.* 2002;12:99–105.

28. Dunn AL, Marcus BH, Kampert JB, Garcia ME, Kohl HW 3rd, Blair SN. Comparison of lifestyle and structured interventions to increase physical activity and cardiorespiratory fitness: a randomized trial. *JAMA.* 1999;281:327–334.

29. Effects of physical activity counseling in primary care. *JAMA.* 2001;286:677–687.

30. Institute of Medicine. *Dietary Reference Intakes for Energy, Carbohydrate, Fiber, Fat, Fatty Acids, Cholesterol, Protein, and Amino Acids* (prepublication version). Washington, DC: National Academies Press; 2002.
31. International Association for the Study of Obesity. *Obesity Newsletter.* 2002;4:14–15.

PART B. Practical Applications

Ruth Ann Carpenter, MS, RD

Practical Approaches to Increasing Physical Activity

In the past many clinicians, including registered dietitians, were trained to refer their clients to exercise physiologists or other exercise specialists for exercise counseling. Although this remains a good practice in some instances, the convergence of several new developments in health promotion has made it important, if not imperative, for all health professionals working with overweight and obese clients to provide physical activity guidance. As described in the Overview section of this chapter, recent research has shown that moderate amounts of physical activity provide significant health benefits, regardless of weight status. The body of evidence and the ensuing public health recommendations expand the options that health professionals can use to promote physical activity.

In addition, the increasing prevalence of obesity suggests that it will take a concerted effort of all health professionals—physicians, dietitians, exercise physiologists, nurses, health educators, and others—to help stem this disturbing trend. Research is leading to evidenced-based physical activity interventions that can be delivered by non-exercise professionals. Studies at The Cooper Institute and at Brown University have shown that a lifestyle approach to physical activity is just as effective as, and is more cost-effective than, a structured exercise program to improve physical fitness, physical activity, and many cardiovascular risk factors (1,2).

Given these recent developments and the fact that physical activity is essential for long-term weight management, the time is right for registered dietitians and other health professionals to provide physical activity guidance as part of a comprehensive approach to treating overweight and obese clients. This section will (1) provide examples of how to help clients implement public health recommendations for physical activity; (2) review methods of physical activity assessment; and (3) address several exercise-related topics that are unique to the severely obese client.

Public Health Guidelines

There are three components of the American College of Sports Medicine/ Centers for Disease Prevention and Control (ACSM/CDC) recommendation for physical activity: intensity, duration, and frequency. The bottom line is that the harder, longer, and more frequently one exercises, the more calories one burns. It should be noted that, although increasing energy expenditure is a primary focus for physical activity's role in weight management, regular moderate-intensity physical activity provides significant health benefits, regardless of weight loss.

Physical Activity: How Intense?

Although any amount of physical activity is better than none, current recommendations emphasize doing at least moderate-intensity activity. Exercise physiologists classify this as any activity that requires 3 to 6 metabolic equivalents (METs) of energy expenditure or 3 to 6 times more than resting intensity. This is equivalent to walking a mile in 15 to 20 minutes—a brisk walk for most individuals. As a professional recommending exercise, the clinician may find it helpful to go to a local high school track and experience what walking a mile in 15 to 20 minutes feels like. An accurate description and demonstration of moderate-intensity activity can be beneficial for the client.

Walking is not the only physical activity that can qualify as moderate in intensity. Box 6B.1 lists other moderate-intensity activities. Note that most activities do not require a gym membership or special exercise equipment.

Does this mean that overweight clients should not exercise at more vigorous levels? Not necessarily. A major advantage of vigorous activity is that

---

Box 6B.1.   Moderate-Intensity Activities

Bicycling, 10 mph	Vigorous vacuuming
Dancing	Sweeping
Hiking	Tai chi
Gardening	Table tennis
Golfing (without a cart)	Washing and waxing a car
Raking leaves	

it burns calories at a higher rate than moderate-intensity activities. However, many weight management clients are inactive and have low fitness levels. This makes it difficult to partake in vigorous activities for very long or without significant risk of injury or burnout. In addition, many vigorous activities require special equipment or instruction (eg, aerobics dance classes, weight training). Quite importantly, taking part in vigorous activity would require some overweight clients to obtain a physician's clearance. Therefore, it is best to help clients to simply start moving, while building up to moderate-intensity activities. In time, as their fitness level improves and their exercise interests expand, you can encourage them to increase the level and length of activity. For clients who are capable of and interested in vigorous activity at the outset of treatment, consider recommending a personal trainer, fitness center, or exercise physiologist who can help with their fitness and exercise training goals.

Physical Activity: How Often?

The public health recommendation for physical activity states that people should be active on most, preferably all, days of the week. For a client doing moderate-intensity activities, this means 5 or more days a week; if an individual is doing vigorous-intensity activity, 3 to 5 days per week is sufficient. The important point is that clients embrace the concept that, to recognize the benefits, especially weight management benefits, physical activity must be regular.

Physical Activity: How Long?

Individuals vary greatly in the amount of exercise needed to prevent weight gain and the amount needed to keep weight off once it is lost. Most studies suggest that at least 30 minutes a day of moderate-intensity activity will provide health benefits. However, more time (ie, 60 minutes or more per day of moderate-intensity activities or less than 60 minutes per day of vigorous-intensity activities) is needed to help control the battle of the bulge.

For most people, overweight or not, exercising 30 to 60+ minutes each day seems daunting. That is why it is important to inform clients that they do not need to get all their daily physical activity in one exercise session. Research now shows that people can obtain similar health and fitness benefits either by accumulating physical activity throughout the day or by exercising in one single exercise session. One study demonstrated that obese women who completed four 10-minute bouts of activity, 5 days a week, ended up with more minutes of moderate activity—and lost more weight—than women who were instructed to complete one 40-minute bout of exercise 5 days a week (3). The bottom line is to help clients to identify ways in which they can build physical activities into their daily routine. Some clients will be able to accomplish one long bout of physical activity each day. Others will need to find ways to do enough short (5 minutes or more) bouts of moderate-intensity activity to reach the goal of 30 minutes or more per day.

Lifestyle Physical Activity

The current public health recommendations for physical activity remove many barriers (eg, lack of time, don't like to sweat, don't like sports) to being more active. Still, clients will need help to find individualized, creative ways to introduce more physical activity into their lifestyle. One way to do this is to ask clients to identify how they can take normally sedentary activities and add activity to them. For example, many clients spend a good portion of their day on the telephone. To increase this lifestyle activity, one client began using a cordless telephone and walked up and down the corridor outside his office as he was taking care of business. Likewise, a soccer mom started walking around her daughter's practice field instead of sitting on the sidelines talking with the other moms. Yet another client used a home exercise bike during TV commercials. In 2 hours of prime-time programs, she accumulated more than 30 minutes of activity. Also, encourage clients to replace sedentary activities with more active pursuits. One client started cycling to work several times a week. A volunteer at the local animal shelter asked to be switched from the receptionist's desk to walking the dogs.

Building small bouts of activity into a daily routine is one part of lifestyle physical activity. Another important aspect of lifestyle physical activity is the development of life management skills that are necessary to make physical activity a regular part of daily living. These cognitive and behavioral skills enable clients to make behavior change relevant to their particular lifestyle and help them to cope with the many challenges of becoming more active. Teaching clients these strategies is nothing new to the registered dietitian. For example, Table 6B.1 compares how different cognitive and behavior change skills can be applied to both diet and physical activity.

Increasing physical activity may make only modest contributions to weight loss, but being active is important in the prevention of weight regain after weight loss. Teaching lifestyle management skills helps set the foundation for a lifetime of physical activity.

Steps to Providing Dietary Guidance

To implement a physical activity plan for overweight and obese clients, their readiness for physical activity will need to be assessed. Then, treatment guidelines can be adapted to the client's interests, abilities, and readiness to change.

Table 6B.1. Applications of Lifestyle Skills to Changing Dietary and Physical Activity Behaviors

Lifestyle Skill	*Dietary Application*	*Physical Activity Application*
Self-monitoring	• Food records	• Physical activity behavior logs • Periodic fitness assessments
Goal setting	• Reduced-calorie intake • Balanced diet	• Increased calorie expenditure
Reward setting	• Tied to healthy eating goals	• Tied to physical activity goals
Social support	• People to help with healthy shopping and cooking tasks • People to encourage healthy eating habits	• People with whom to exercise and to help with life activities so client can have time to be active
Stimulus control	• Removing empty-calorie items from counters, cupboards, and refrigerators	• Keeping walking shoes at office, in car, in travel bag
Cognitive restructuring	• All foods can fit (eliminating all-or-none thinking)	• Any activity is better than no activity
Increasing healthy opportunities	• Finding heart-healthy restaurants • Trying new low-fat food • Taking healthful cooking classes	• Finding parks, recreation centers, trails, activity clubs in local community • Putting home exercise equipment in conspicuous place
Relapse prevention	• Planning ahead for high-calorie or inappropriate eating situations • Positive-thinking strategies to get back on track after a lapse • Cognitive skills to cope with urges to eat unhealthful foods	• Planning ahead for disruptions to activity plans (eg, time constraints, weather, injury) • Positive-thinking strategies to get back on track after a lapse • Cognitive skills to cope with urges to skip doing physical activity

Assessment

There are three types of assessments that can be useful in helping overweight and obese clients prepare physical activity plans. One is the assessment of a client's current physical fitness status. Traditional exercise interventions use a measured fitness level as the base on which a structured exercise prescription is developed. The lifestyle approach suggested earlier in this section does not require a baseline fitness level. Still, periodic fitness assessments can provide useful feedback to the client and the clinician on the effects of an increase in physical activity level. Fitness assessment tests are normally administered by trained clinicians, exercise physiologists, or other experts and, as such, are beyond the scope of this section. However, if the client is interested in obtaining this information, refer him or her to a qualified exercise professional, such as a certified personal trainer or exercise physiologist.

Two assessments that should be administered to all clients are an exercise preparticipation screening and an assessment of motivational readiness to become more physically active.

PAR-Q

The Physical Activity Readiness Questionnaire (PAR-Q) is one way to discern who should get a doctor's clearance to exercise (see Figure 6B.1) (4). The PAR-Q is very specific about the steps that should be taken before starting an exercise program. It is best to administer the PAR-Q during a client's initial visit. If, after administering the PAR-Q, it appears safe for the client to start exercising, proceed with the motivational readiness assessment process. However, if the client's answers to the questions indicate that he or she should see a doctor, then delay discussing physical activity any further until the client obtains written clearance from the physician to start exercising.

If a client for whom the screening protocol recommends a doctor's clearance before beginning activity is not able or is unwilling to see a doctor, refrain from discussing physical activity changes. Address the benefits of physical activity, but do not work with the client to devise a specific physical activity plan.

Assessing Motivational Readiness

Because an individual may be physically ready to start exercising does not mean that he or she will start. Motivational readiness plays a big role in a person's willingness to listen to messages about physical activity and to start the process of becoming more active. Behavior change is a very complex process, but the Transtheoretical Model, or Stages of Change (SOC) Model, provides a useful tool for clinicians to be more effective in their physical

Physical Activity Readiness
Questionnaire - PAR-Q
(revised 2002)

PAR-Q & YOU

(A Questionnaire for People Aged 15 to 69)

Regular physical activity is fun and healthy, and increasingly more people are starting to become more active every day. Being more active is very safe for most people. However, some people should check with their doctor before they start becoming much more physically active.

If you are planning to become much more physically active than you are now, start by answering the seven questions in the box below. If you are between the ages of 15 and 69, the PAR-Q will tell you if you should check with your doctor before you start. If you are over 69 years of age, and you are not used to being very active, check with your doctor.

Common sense is your best guide when you answer these questions. Please read the questions carefully and answer each one honestly: check YES or NO.

YES	NO		
☐	☐	1.	Has your doctor ever said that you have a heart condition <u>and</u> that you should only do physical activity recommended by a doctor?
☐	☐	2.	Do you feel pain in your chest when you do physical activity?
☐	☐	3.	In the past month, have you had chest pain when you were not doing physical activity?
☐	☐	4.	Do you lose your balance because of dizziness or do you ever lose consciousness?
☐	☐	5.	Do you have a bone or joint problem (for example, back, knee or hip) that could be made worse by a change in your physical activity?
☐	☐	6.	Is your doctor currently prescribing drugs (for example, water pills) for your blood pressure or heart condition?
☐	☐	7.	Do you know of <u>any other reason</u> why you should not do physical activity?

If you answered

YES to one or more questions

Talk with your doctor by phone or in person BEFORE you start becoming much more physically active or BEFORE you have a fitness appraisal. Tell your doctor about the PAR-Q and which questions you answered YES.

- You may be able to do any activity you want — as long as you start slowly and build up gradually. Or, you may need to restrict your activities to those which are safe for you. Talk with your doctor about the kinds of activities you wish to participate in and follow his/her advice.
- Find out which community programs are safe and helpful for you.

NO to all questions

If you answered NO honestly to <u>all</u> PAR-Q questions, you can be reasonably sure that you can:
- start becoming much more physically active — begin slowly and build up gradually. This is the safest and easiest way to go.
- take part in a fitness appraisal – this is an excellent way to determine your basic fitness so that you can plan the best way for you to live actively. It is also highly recommended that you have your blood pressure evaluated. If your reading is over 144/94, talk with your doctor before you start becoming much more physically active.

→

DELAY BECOMING MUCH MORE ACTIVE:
- if you are not feeling well because of a temporary illness such as a cold or a fever – wait until you feel better; or
- if you are or may be pregnant – talk to your doctor before you start becoming more active.

PLEASE NOTE: If your health changes so that you then answer YES to any of the above questions, tell your fitness or health professional. Ask whether you should change your physical activity plan.

<u>Informed Use of the PAR-Q</u>: The Canadian Society for Exercise Physiology, Health Canada, and their agents assume no liability for persons who undertake physical activity, and if in doubt after completing this questionnaire, consult your doctor prior to physical activity.

No changes permitted. You are encouraged to photocopy the PAR-Q but only if you use the entire form.

NOTE: If the PAR-Q is being given to a person before he or she participates in a physical activity program or a fitness appraisal, this section may be used for legal or administrative purposes.

"I have read, understood and completed this questionnaire. Any questions I had were answered to my full satisfaction."

NAME _____

SIGNATURE _____ DATE _____

SIGNATURE OF PARENT _____ WITNESS _____
or GUARDIAN (for participants under the age of majority)

Note: This physical activity clearance is valid for a maximum of 12 months from the date it is completed and becomes invalid if your condition changes so that you would answer YES to any of the seven questions.

CSEP © Canadian Society for Exercise Physiology   Supported by: ▮✦| Health Canada Santé Canada

Figure 6B.1. Physical Activity Readiness Questionnaire (PAR-Q).
Source: Physical Activity Readiness Questionnaire (PAR-Q) © 2002. Reprinted with permission from the Canadian Society of Exercise Physiology. http://www.csep.ca/forms.asp.

activity guidance. The SOC Model posits that people move through different stages in the process of adopting a new health behavior (5). People advance through the stages by applying different behavioral and cognitive skills. Table 6B.2 lists the five stages of readiness, typical characteristics of people in each physical activity readiness stage, and appropriate goals and actions for counseling clients in each stage.

The practitioner's goal should be to help a client move from one stage to the next. For example, it may be inappropriate to tell a person in the precontemplation stage that he or she should start exercising—they are simply not ready to change. Instead, the goal should be to get a precontemplator to start thinking about being more active (ie, to move to the contemplation stage). Be prepared to help the client understand the many benefits of physical activity, to dispel myths about exercise, and to help the client identify any exercise barriers. These actions are likely to help the client take the next step (ie, thinking about being more active) in the journey to reaching the maintenance stage. Remember, different clients are going to be in different stages. Tailor recommendations to each client's motivational readiness. A "one size fits all" exercise recommendation will not be helpful to most clients.

What stage is a client in? Often simply listening to what a client says about physical activity can be very revealing. "I don't exercise now and I don't see what good it is going to do me" is something a precontemplator might say. A person in the preparation stage might say, "I got a new pair of walking shoes and I am going to start exercising on Monday." "I've been doing at least 30 minutes of moderate exercise at least 5 days a week for the last 3 months, but I am getting bored," might be something you would hear from a person in the action stage.

Figure 6B.2 shows another way to determine a person's readiness to become more physically active (6). This simple flow diagram is easy to administer. Be sure that clients fully comprehend the first box. Some clients do not give themselves credit for the smaller bouts of moderate activity (eg, walking the dog, walking from the subway to the office, raking leaves) that they get throughout the day. At the same time, many people have a tendency to overestimate their activity level.

Neither the professional nor the client should expect a linear progression through the stages of change. Behavior change is often a process of two steps forward, one step back. In other words, lapses are to be expected. Advise clients that lapses are part of the learning process. On the positive side, if clients experience lapses during treatment, help them (1) to identify what triggered the lapse and how to deal with the trigger in the future and (2) to develop cognitive skills to accept a lapse as a temporary setback and to use positive thinking skills to prevent the lapse from leading to a total collapse of the physical activity adoption effort. When a client lapses to an earlier

Table 6B.2. Characteristics, Goals, and Actions for Different Stages of Readiness to Change Physical Activity Level

Stage of Readiness	Characteristics of Stage	Stage-appropriate Goal and Action
Precontemplation	• Doesn't think about being more active • Doesn't recognize personal benefits of being active; may have tried and failed in the past • Has lots of barriers (real and perceived) • Has very low exercise self-efficacy (ie, lack of self-confidence)	*Goal: Move to Contemplation* 1. Discuss the benefits of regular physical activity (ie, weight management, CHD risk reduction, reduced stress, bone health, diabetes risk reduction) 2. Identify the client's personal barriers 3. Educate about moderate-intensity activity and accumulating physical activity 4. Encourage client to think about physical activity, not necessarily to do more activity
Contemplation	• Thinks about being more active but doesn't do anything • Knows some benefits but has many barriers • Doesn't know how to get started	*Goal: Move to Preparation* Numbers 1–3 above, plus have client: 1. Commit to doing a few 2-minute walks each week, gradually building up to several per day 2. Begin to address major barriers 3. Identify how client can turn sedentary activities into more active ones (eg, walking at the park while children have soccer practice)
Preparation	• Intends to become more active in the near future or to do some physical activity but not enough to achieve public health goal • Can get started but can't stay with it • More benefits but still has a lot of barriers	*Goal: Move to Action* All of the above, plus have client: 1. Set short- and long-term goals and rewards 2. Recruit support 3. Track thoughts about activity or actual activity (ie, minutes, steps, distance) 4. Congratulate client on doing something

(continues)

Table 6B.2. (Continued)

Stage of Readiness	Characteristics of Stage	Stage-appropriate Goal and Action
Action	• Achieving public health goal but for less than 6 months • Most use of cognitive and behavioral skills (ie, goal-setting, self-monitoring, social support) • At the greatest risk of relapse • Knows or has experienced some physical activity benefits	*Goal: Move to Maintenance* All of the above, plus have client: 1. Plan for lapses and high-risk situations 2. Identify physical activity resources in the community 3. Try new activities 4. Track activity (steps, minutes, distance) 5. Set new short-term and long-term goals 6. Praise client's progress and commitment
Maintenance	• Achieves public health goal for longer than 6 months • Very high exercise self-efficacy • Has realized many physical activity benefits • Physical activity is a personal value	*Goal: Stay in Maintenance* All of the above, plus have client: 1. Cite keys for personal success 2. Help others to become more active 3. Identify alternative physical activities 4. Determine whether or not he or she is ready to add other or more vigorous activities to program

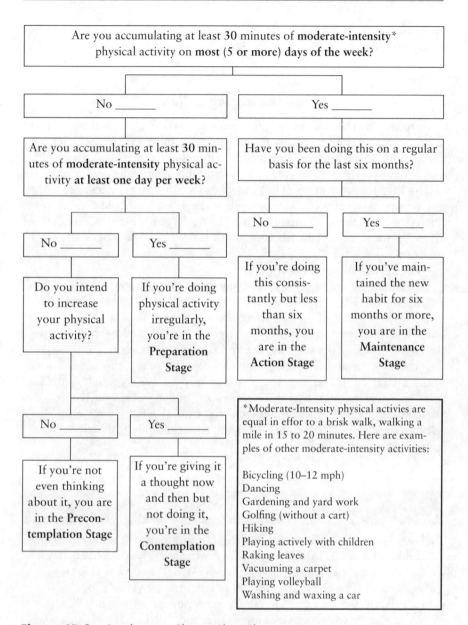

Are you accumulating at least **30** minutes of **moderate-intensity***
physical activity on **most (5 or more) days of the week?**

No _____   **Yes** _____

Are you accumulating at least **30** minutes of **moderate-intensity** physical activity **at least one day per week?**

Have you been doing this on a regular basis for the last six months?

No _____   **Yes** _____

If you're doing this consistantly but less than six months, you are in the **Action Stage**

If you've maintained the new habit for six months or more, you are in the **Maintenance Stage**

No _____   **Yes** _____

Do you intend to increase your physical activity?

If you're doing physical activity irregularly, you're in the **Preparation Stage**

No _____   **Yes** _____

If you're not even thinking about it, you are in the **Precontemplation Stage**

If you're giving it a thought now and then but not doing it, you're in the **Contemplation Stage**

*Moderate-Intensity physical activies are equal in effor to a brisk walk, walking a mile in 15 to 20 minutes. Here are examples of other moderate-intensity activities:

Bicycling (10–12 mph)
Dancing
Gardening and yard work
Golfing (without a cart)
Hiking
Playing actively with children
Raking leaves
Vacuuming a carpet
Playing volleyball
Washing and waxing a car

Figure 6B.2.   Readiness to Change Flow Chart
Reprinted by permission, from SN Blair et al, 2001. *Active Living Every Day* (Champaign, Ill: Human Kinetics), 9.

stage of readiness, return to the strategies that helped the client move forward initially.

Implementing a Plan

The American Dietetic Association has provided guidelines that set forth comprehensive clinical treatment procedures in the areas of assessment, intervention, and self-management training (including physical activity intervention), plans for follow-up, and communication with other relevant health care team members. The guidelines recommend six encounters, during 6 months, with periodic follow-up as needed. These guidelines are currently part of the Commission on Dietetic Registration's "Certificate of Training in Adult Weight Management" course (7). Table 6B.3 shows the recommended actions and practical counseling strategies related to physical activity at each of the six encounters.

Depending on whether it is an initial visit or a follow-up visit, a typical weight-management counseling session may last 20 to 60 minutes. This is a limited amount of time to cover the many tasks associated with assessment and intervention in nutrition, physical activity, and behavioral areas. In addition, clinicians who do not specialize in exercise may not be comfortable talking about exercise issues. Likewise, many clients tend to be more interested in learning about dietary approaches to weight reduction than in learning about exercise (ie, they are in early stages of readiness to change). Be aware of these roadblocks to physical activity intervention and work to help your overweight clients improve their physical activity behaviors as well as their eating habits.

Case Study. Dora

Dora is a 47-year-old woman living in upstate New York with three children (ages 20, 15, 12 years), a husband who drives a delivery truck for a national overnight shipping company, and two large dogs. Dora works part-time (3 days a week) as an accounting clerk at a local newspaper publisher near her home. A good portion of her day is spent shuttling her two youngest children to school and sports activities. She also volunteers 2 days per month at a local nursing home. Dora is 64 inches tall and weighs 190 pounds (BMI = 33). Her weight history indicates a gradual increase in weight since high school, when she weighed 140 pounds. She started gaining weight with the birth of the children—about 10 to 12 pounds with each child. At times, she has lost 10 to 15 pounds on various fad diets but always gained it back

Table 6B.3. Physical Activity Recommendations for Medical Nutrition Therapy Protocol for Weight Management

Encounter	Interval Between Visits	Physical Activity Recommendations	Practical Application
1	Within 30 d of referral	• Assess client's readiness to learn • Assess physical activity pattern (attitude toward physical activity, personal history, knowledge about physical activity) • Mutually establish short- and long-term goals for physical activity	• If not previously cleared for exercise, administer PAR-Q • Ask about client's personal barriers to, and potential benefits of, being more active • Administer "Readiness to Change" flow sheet • Set goals according to client's readiness stage (see Figure 6B.2) • Educate client about physical activity's role in weight loss and, especially, maintenance of weight loss
2, 3, and 4	2–4 wk	• Assess client's adherence to and comprehension of physical activity. Compare to expected outcomes and goals. • Reinforce or modify life skills strategies • Reinforce or modify mutual short- and long-term goals for physical activity	• Review physical activity logs* • Help client use problem-solving mindset to address one or two physical activity barriers • Re-administer "Readiness to Change" flow sheet every 4 wk • Set goals according to client's readiness stage (see Figure 6B.2) • Reinforce role of physical activity in weight loss and prevention of weight regain
5 and 6	4–6 wk	• Assess client's adherence to and comprehension of physical activity. Compare to expected outcomes and goals. • Reinforce or modify life skills strategies • Reinforce or modify mutual short- and long-term goals for physical activity • Discuss lapse and relapse prevention.	• Review physical activity logs* • Help client use problem-solving mindset to address one or two physical activity barriers • Re-administer "Readiness to Change" flow sheet • Set goals according to client's readiness stage (see Figure 6B.2) • Reinforce role of physical activity in weight loss and prevention of weight regain • Have client make plans for coping with high-risk situations (eg, holidays, vacations, travel, family emergencies, bad weather)

*Logging thoughts about physical activity is a good self-monitoring skill for people who have not yet begun to be more active.

plus more. Dora has borderline hypertension and normal fasting glucose and triglyceride levels. Lipitor has brought her blood cholesterol levels into an acceptable range. She is not using any other medication on a regular basis. Dora comes to you on the advice of a friend who is a client. Your nutrition assessment indicates that she eats excessive fat and sugar calories, mostly from snack foods. Jelly beans are a "stress food" for her. She lacks adequate fruit intake but does "pretty well" in the other food groups. She has indicated that she is "really ready" to start eating better. As for physical activity, she loved tap and jazz dance as a child but did not participate in any organized activities as an adolescent or young adult. She attempted aerobics classes but found them strenuous and inconvenient.

As she has gotten older, Dora's knees have begun to hurt more, especially while climbing hills and stairs. Her doctor has told her that it is probably the beginning of arthritis and that physical activity and weight loss would likely improve her symptoms. Dora enjoys being outside except when it is really cold or wet, which in upstate New York is a big part of the year.

Questions to Consider

- Does Dora need to see a physician before you start working with her on her physical activity?
- Dora is likely in what stage of readiness to change?
- What seems to be her barriers to physical activity?
- What might be the benefits she could gain from being active?

Using the principles described in this chapter, here are clinical guidelines for providing physical activity guidance to Dora during a six-encounter weight-management program.

Encounter #1—March 1

Assessment

- Not previously cleared for exercise.
- Not capable or interested in doing vigorous activities; willing to try moderate-intensity activities.
- Cleared for moderate-intensity activities using PAR-Q instrument.
- Barriers to activity: time, family responsibilities, doesn't like to sweat, uncomfortable wearing exercise clothes.
- Perceived personal benefits: weight loss.
- Stage of readiness to change physical activity: Contemplation.

- Enjoyed dance as a child but was not active as an adolescent or young adult; aerobics classes were too strenuous; enjoys walking in neighborhood; doesn't like cold; knows exercise is important.

Intervention

- Educate about physical activity's role in weight loss and, especially, maintenance of weight loss.
- Educate on the personally relevant benefits of moderate-intensity physical activity, especially weight management, stress management, energy enhancement, and cardiovascular disease risk reduction.
- Educate on accumulation of activity throughout the day.
- Short-term goal (next 2 weeks): keep a log of thoughts about physical activity and actual physical activity; do one brisk 2-minute walk per day for 10 of the next 14 days.
- Long-term goal (in 5 months)—accumulate at least 30 minutes of moderate-intensity activity 5 or more days per week.

Encounter #2—March 15

Assessment

- Log indicated increased number of thoughts about physical activity in second week; did not log activity time.
- Achieved goal for 2-minute walks on 5 days; has a hard time remembering to think about being more active.
- Family responsibilities often upset her physical activity plans.
- Purchased comfortable walking shoes.

Intervention

- Dora brainstormed about ways to fit physical activity into family time (walk around soccer field, go dancing with husband on "date night," walk the dog after dinner).
- Reinforced role of physical activity in weight loss and prevention of weight regain.
- Short-term goals (next 2 weeks): keep a log of thoughts about physical activity and actual physical activity; do one brisk 2-minute walk per day for 10 of the next 14 days; do at least one activity with family that is active.
- Long-term goal (in 5 months): accumulate at least 30 minutes of moderate-intensity activity 5 or more days per week.

Encounter # 3—March 30

Assessment

- Continuing to increase the number of thoughts about physical activity; logged activity for 2 weeks.
- Achieved goal for 2-minute walks on 10 days; family walked to church together 1 day (15 minutes each way); walked around ball field during son's game.
- Knees hurt during walk to church.
- Feels more confident about ability to fit in short bouts of activity; wants to do more.
- Administration of "Readiness to Change" flow sheet shows Dora is still in Contemplation.

Intervention

- Discussed need to be more gradual in becoming more active, to prevent pain and injury.
- Encouraged Dora to identify sedentary activities that she does and ways to make them more active.
- Short-term goals (next 4 weeks): keep a log of thoughts about physical activity and actual physical activity; take two brisk 5-minute walks per day for at least 5 days each week; turn one sedentary activity into an opportunity for activity.
- Long-term goal (in 5 months): accumulate at least 30 minutes of moderate-intensity activity 5 or more days per week.

Encounter # 4—May 1

Assessment

- Logged activity for 3 of 4 weeks; accumulated more than 30 minutes on 5 days.
- Achieved goal for 5-minute walks (2 per day) for 4 weeks; walked instead of drove to neighbor's for monthly bridge game; continued walking at soccer games 15 minutes, twice a week (got two other mothers to walk with her); walks dogs for 10 to 15 minutes several times a week
- Has a hard time fitting in walks on days that she works at the newspaper publisher.
- Beginning to feel less tired when walking; has a little more energy, though she is getting a little bored with walking.
- Administration of "Readiness to Change" flow sheet shows Dora has moved to Preparation stage.

Intervention

- Encouraged Dora to increase number of 5-minute walks; pointed out how close she was to reaching long-term goal of at least 30 minutes on most days; encouraged her to find new activities or people with whom to do activities.
- Short-term goals (next 4 weeks): keep a log of physical activity; do two brisk 10-minute walks per day for at least 5 days per week; walk to part-time job (20 minutes) at least 2 days per week.
- Long-term goal (in 5 months): accumulate at least 30 minutes of moderate-intensity activity 5 or more days per week.

Encounter #5—June 1

Assessment

- Logged activity for first 2 weeks only: stress at work, lost logging sheets, and end-of-school-year activities prevented logging.
- Unsure what, if any, goals she met since last visit; she did think about being active and fit in some walks; did not walk to job.
- Feeling "stressed out"; having a hard time making time for herself.
- Very discouraged and ready to give up.
- Administration of "Readiness to Change" flow sheet shows that Dora has lapsed back to Contemplation stage.

Intervention

- Praised her for doing what she could under the circumstances.
- Discussed the inevitability of lapses; described importance of positive thinking to prevent a lapse from becoming a relapse; encouraged Dora to analyze what contributed to the lapse and to learn from it.
- Emphasized the importance of physical activity in managing stress.
- Introduced the step counter as a simple method for logging activity; demonstrated its use.
- Short-term goals (next 6 weeks): keep a log of steps taken each day; increase average daily number of steps by 200 to 500 steps each week after first week; build back up to doing at least two brisk 10-minute walks per day for at least 5 days per week; walk to part-time job (20 minutes) at least 2 days per week; find ways to be active with family.
- Long-term goal (in 5 months): accumulate at least 30 minutes of moderate-intensity activity 5 or more days per week.

Encounter #6—July 15

Assessment

- Client loved step counter. Averaged 6,300 steps the first week; increased 500+ daily steps per week and is now averaging nearly 10,000 steps per day.
- Administration of "Readiness to Change" flow sheet shows that Dora has progressed to the Action stage.
- Feeling more confident after recovering from her lapse; not as stressed out.
- Blood pressure has decreased, and her knees do not hurt as much.

Intervention

- Praised her for reaching her long-term goal.
- Reviewed the strategies that worked best for her. Reminded her that she will need to keep using these strategies to maintain her activity level.
- Reminded her about the long-term benefits of physical activity, regardless of weight loss, and the importance of activity for long-term weight management.
- Encouraged her to increase daily activity time gradually to 60 minutes or to begin to include more vigorous activities by trying new activities.
- Made plans for maintaining activity level when weather turns cold and icy (eg, get comfortable, safe boots to wear so she can still walk to work, check ads for used treadmills or stationary bikes, walk at shopping mall, learn to cross-country ski).
- Short-term goals (next 4 weeks): increase activity time by 10 minutes per day; go dancing with husband at least 3 times per month; find new physical activities to enjoy.
- Long-term goal (in 6 months): accumulate at least 45 to 60 minutes of moderate-intensity activity 5 or more days per week.

Special Topics in Physical Activity for Weight Management

Role of Strength Training in Weight Management

This chapter has focused primarily on moderate-intensity lifestyle activities as the preferred type of physical activity. Moderate-intensity activities (1) can provide weight management and health benefits; (2) can remove the barrier of getting a medical clearance before exercising for many clients; (3) does not require special equipment or instruction and can be incorporated into many daily routines; and (4) is appropriate for those who are not physically fit enough to do vigorous activities. Still, it is important to recognize the role that strength or resistance training (considered a vigorous activity) can have in promoting health and maintaining weight.

First, as individuals lose weight, there is often a slight loss of muscle tissue. Since muscle is very metabolically active—that is, it burns calories all day long—muscle loss can lead to a decline in total daily energy expenditure, and hence, to difficulties in preventing weight regain. Any physical activity will help to attenuate this loss, but strength training may be the most effective exercise for minimizing muscle loss. Second, new studies suggest that resistance training may have health benefits independent of total physical activity level (8). Third, strength training can improve an individual's ability to perform daily tasks, such as carrying groceries, climbing stairs, getting off a sofa or chair, and general mobility. Finally, strength training can tone muscles, thus reducing the appearance of sagging skin that some individuals experience after losing weight.

From a practical perspective, strength training is a great complement to aerobic activity. It is likely that most obese clients will not be ready for strength training activities at the beginning of treatment. However, as they gain fitness experience and more confidence in their ability to be active, you can recommend strength training as another important component of a healthy lifestyle. Since strength training is considered a vigorous activity, review the need for medical clearance.

There are many tools that can help clients improve their strength and fitness, including resistance bands, hand weights, calisthenics (ie, using own body weight as resistance), weight machines, and free weights. Each of these methods requires some instruction. Some equipment may come with directions for use. In the absence of specialized training in this area, it is best to refer clients to certified personal trainers or to exercise physiologists for strength training instruction.

Issues for the Severely Obese

Although being physically active is healthy at any size, the severely obese client may have special concerns. Orthopedic problems, body image issues, health risk factors, balance problems, and chafing can be roadblocks to physical activity for many obese clients. Some obese clients may want to wait until they have lost weight before they start increasing their activity. Be mindful not to ignore the topic of physical activity with these clients. Instead, use the strategies outlined in Table 6B.2 for precontemplators and contemplators.

For severely obese clients who do want to begin some activity, here are suggestions for coping with common problems they may face. Also, many of the resources listed in Chapter 10: Patient and Professional Resources are specifically relevant to this population.

- Orthopedic or balance problems: non–weight-bearing activities, such as water exercise classes, chair aerobics, and recumbent stationary cycling, are good options.
- Body image issues: suggest videos they can do at home (see resource section at the end of this chapter); seek out exercise facilities or instructors who are sensitive to large-size clients.
- Health risk factors: use the assessment guidelines in this chapter to guide you regarding the need to seek medical clearance before increasing physical activity level; periodically check risk-factor status to determine whether adjustments to medication are needed.
- Chafing: encourage a very gradual increase in activity; tight clothing will minimize chafing better than loose clothing; keep areas that rub as dry as possible (talcum or baby powder can help) or use a lubricant, such as bag balm, petroleum jelly, or other lubricating gel.

The important thing to remember when working with severely obese clients is that, although they may have some issues that require special consideration, they should be treated as you would treat any other overweight client—that is, match your recommendations to their readiness to change, their physical activity interests, and their abilities.

Final Note

Remember, even if your clients do not lose any weight during their treatment, if they increase their physical activity level, then they are very likely to be healthier than when they started. Below are a few final preparations that you can make to provide physical activity guidance to your overweight clients.

- Complete the PAR-Q form yourself so that you know when a referral to the doctor is necessary.
- Complete the "Readiness to Change" form, to assess your readiness to change your own physical activity level.
- Get a feel for what moderate-intensity feels like by mapping out a 1-mile distance on a flat surface and walking it in 15 to 20 minutes.
- Develop a referral list of exercise physiologists or personal trainers who are capable of working with overweight clients who want to do more vigorous exercise.

References

1. Dunn AL, Marcus BH, Kampert JB, Garcia ME, Kohl HW 3rd, Blair SN. Comparison of lifestyle and structured interventions to increase physical activity and cardiorespiratory fitness: a randomized trial. *JAMA.* 1999;281:327–334.
2. Sevick MA, Dunn AL, Morrow MS, Marcus BH, Chen GJ, Blair SN. Cost-effectiveness of lifestyle and structured exercise interventions in sedentary adults: results of project ACTIVE. *Am J Prev Med.* 2000;19:1–8.
3. Jakicic JM, Wing RR, Butler BA, Robertson RJ. Prescribing exercise in multiple short bouts versus one continuous bout: effects on adherence, cardiorespiratory fitness, and weight loss in overweight women. *Int J Obes Relat Metab Disord.* 1995;19:893–901.
4. Physical Activity Readiness Questionnaire (PAR-Q). Canadian Society of Exercise Physiology Web site. Available at: http://www.csep.ca/forms.asp. Accessed: June 25, 2003.
5. Prochaska JO, Norcross JC, DiClemente CC. *Changing for Good: A Revolutionary Six-Stage Program for Overcoming Bad Habits and Moving Your Life Positively Forward.* New York, NY: Avon Books; 1995.
6. Blair SN, Dunn A, Marcus B, Carpenter R, Jaret P. *Active Living Every Day.* Champaign, Ill: Human Kinetics; 2001.
7. American Dietetic Association. Weight management (adult) medical nutrition therapy protocol CD-ROM. In: *The American Dietetic Association MNT Evidence-Based Guides for Practice CD-ROMs.* Chicago, Ill: American Dietetic Association; 2003.
8. Tanasescu M, Leitzmann MF, Rimm EB, Willett WC, Stampfer MJ, Hu FB. Exercise type and intensity in relation to coronary heart disease in men. *JAMA.* 2002;288:1994–2000.

Chapter 7

Pharmacological Treatment

PART A. Overview

Jonathan A. Waitman, MD, and Louis J. Aronne, MD

Given the increasing prevalence of obesity (1) and the availability of an-tiobesity agents approved for long-term use, health care professionals should be familiar with the basic principles regarding the pharmacotherapy of obesity. Medications are currently indicated in the treatment of obesity for patients with body mass index (BMI) ≥ 30 or BMI ≥ 27 with other risk factors or diseases. The goals of treatment are to reduce weight and, more importantly, to improve the comorbid conditions associated with obesity, such as hyperglycemia, hyperlipidemia, and hypertension. Patients will need assistance in recognizing that obesity is a chronic disease that requires long-term treatment. Patients for whom medications are appropriate should also be educated about the efficacy of the current medications, which, for most, results in approximately a 5% to 10% weight loss. Finally, medications should be used only as an adjunct to healthful lifestyle changes. The purpose of this chapter is to provide a brief overview of the medications that are cur-rently used by physicians to treat obesity.

Medications Approved for Long-term Use

Sibutramine (Meridia) and orlistat (Xenical) are the only medications cur-rently approved for the long-term treatment of obesity (2). Both of these medications have proven efficacy in achieving and maintaining weight loss when compared with placebo (see Tables 7A.1 and 7A.2) (3–17).

Sibutramine (Meridia)

Mechanism.   Sibutramine reduces food intake by inhibiting the reuptake of norepinephrine, dopamine, and serotonin. Table 7A.1 lists representative sibutramine studies that are described below.

Short- and Long-term Weight Loss.   Bray et al evaluated different doses of sibutramine during a 24-week period (3). They found a statistically significant weight loss at all doses (1, 5, 10, 15, 20, and 30 mg) compared with placebo. Wirth and Krause showed that intermittent sibutramine was as effective as continuous sibutramine over a 44-week period (4). Apfelbaum et al studied obese patients (BMI > 30) who consumed very-low-calorie diets for 4 weeks, followed by 1 year of sibutramine vs placebo. A greater percentage of subjects who received sibutramine than those who took the placebo maintained their weight loss at 1 year (5). In the longest study of sibutramine, James et al showed that 18 months after initial weight loss, 43% of the patients maintained ≥ 80% of their original weight loss vs 9% in the placebo group (18). These studies illustrate sibutramine's efficacy as a weight-loss and weight-maintenance agent, and that most weight loss takes place during the first 6 months of treatment.

Special Populations.   McMahon et al (8) and Sramek et al (19) each demonstrated the safety of sibutramine in the treatment of obese patients

Table 7A.1. Randomized Controlled Trials of Sibutramine

Study	Subjects	Study Period	Dose (mg/d)	Placebo Weight Change	Sibutramine Weight Change	P
Bray et al (3)	1,463	24 wk	5	–1.20%	–3.90%	< .05
			10		–6.10%	
			15		–7.40%	
			20		–8.80%	
Wirth and Kraus (4)	1,102	44 wk	15	+0.2%		< .05
Apfelbaum et al (5)	160	1 y	10	+0.5 kg	–5.2 kg	< .04
Cuellar et al (6)	69	6 mo	15	–1.26 kg	–10.27 kg	< .001
Gokcel et al (7)	54	6 mo	20	–0.91 kg	–9.61 kg	< .0001
McMahon et al (8)	220	1 y	20	–0.4 kg	–4.5 kg	< .05
McMahon et al (9)	124	1 y	20	–0.70%	–4.70%	< .05

Table 7A.2.   Randomized Controlled Trials of Orlistat

Study	Number	Study Period	Dose (mg/d)	Placebo Weight Change	Orlistat Weight Change	P
Rossner et al (10)	729	1 y	360	−6.60%	−8.60%	< .001
			180	−6.60%	−9.70%	< .001
Sjostrom et al (11)	743	1 y	360	−6.10%	−10.20%	< .001
Davidson et al (12)	892	2 y	360	−5.81 kg	−8.76 kg	< .001
Finer et al (13)	228	1 y	360	−8.50%	−5.40%	< .016
Hauptman et al (14)	796	1 y	360	−4.14 kg	−7.94 kg	< .01
			180	−4.14 kg	−7.08 kg	< .01
Hollander et al (15)	391	57 wk	360	−4.30%	−6.40%	< .001
Lindgarde (16)	382	1 y	360	−4.60%	−5.90%	< .05
Kelley et al (17)	550	1 y	360	+1.27%	−3.89%	< .001

with well-controlled hypertension. These studies found statistically significant increases in pulse rate, but not blood pressure, in the sibutramine groups. Sibutramine has been proven safe in patients being treated with hypertensive medications (8,9,19) and has been shown to be effective in the treatment of diabetes (20).

Side Effects.   The most frequent side effects associated with sibutramine are dry mouth, anorexia, and insomnia. Patients may experience an increase in blood pressure and pulse, and monitoring of these vital signs should be performed on a monthly basis initially and every 3 months once the patient's weight has stabilized. Although the cardiac effects of the combination of other anorexigenic agents dexfenfluramine and fenfluramine led to the withdrawal of these drugs from the market in 1997, Zannad et al found that 6 months of sibutramine had no significant impact on cardiac dimension, valve function, or electrocardiograms (21).

Orlistat (Xenical)

Mechanism.   Orlistat promotes weight loss by inhibiting gastrointestinal lipases and by decreasing the absorption of fat from the gastrointestinal tract. On average, 120 mg of orlistat taken 3 times per day will decrease fat absorption by 30% (22). Orlistat has been found to be more effective in inhibiting the digestion of solid foods, as opposed to liquids (23). Representative studies are summarized in Table 7A.2 and are described below.

Short- and Long-term Weight Loss.   Rossner et al (10) found that subjects receiving orlistat lost significantly more weight in the first year of treatment, and fewer regained weight during the second year of treatment than those taking placebo. The orlistat group also had greater improvement in their cardiovascular profiles (LDL-C and total cholesterol). Subjects taking orlistat had significantly lower serum levels of vitamins D, E, and beta carotene. However, these decreases are easily treated with oral multivitamin supplementation. Sjostrom et al (11) demonstrated similar weight loss during a 2-year period. Subjects in the orlistat group lost significantly more weight in the first year (10.2% vs 6.1%) and regained half as much weight during the second year.

In another 2-year study, Davidson et al (12) showed that there was less weight regain in patients maintained on the 360-mg-per-day dose of orlistat, as opposed to a 60-mg-per-day dose or placebo. Subjects in the orlistat group also had lower levels of serum glucose and insulin.

Special Populations.   Hollander el al studied obese patients with type 2 diabetes (15). Orlistat resulted in improved glycemic control (blood glucose and HbA1C), and reductions in total cholesterol, LDL-C, triglycerides, and apo-lipoprotein B. Kelley et al showed similar benefits in obese insulin-requiring diabetics (17). Lindgarde examined the impact of orlistat on cardiovascular profiles in obese subjects with at least one of the following: type 2 diabetes, hypercholesterolemia, and hypertension (16). Orlistat use was associated with greater weight loss and reductions in HbA1c, LDL-C, and total cholesterol. LDL-C reduction was found to be greater than the effect of weight loss in those patients with obesity and hypercholesterolemia (24).

Side Effects.   The gastrointestinal side effects of orlistat, including fatty or oily stool, fecal urgency, oily spotting, increased defecation, fecal incontinence, flatus with discharge, and oily evacuation, are the main reasons for discontinuation of therapy. These symptoms are usually mild to moderate and decrease in frequency the longer the medication is continued. Cavaliere et al (25) examined the effect of concomitant use of natural fibers (psyllium mucilloid) on gastrointestinal side effects. Subjects who received the psyllium experienced far fewer symptoms—only 29% of those taking psyllium with orlistat (120 mg tid) had gastrointestinal events compared with 71% of the patients on placebo with orlistat.

Comparative Study.   In the only comparative study of orlistat and sibutramine, Gokcel et al (7) compared the effects of sibutramine (10 mg twice daily) with orlistat (120 mg three times daily) and metformin (850 mg twice daily) in obese females. After 6 months of treatment, all three groups showed significant improvements in lipid profiles, insulin resistance, glucose, and blood pressure. Sibutramine produced a statistically significant ($P < .0001$) greater reduction in BMI (13.6%) when compared with orlistat (9.1%) and metformin (9.9%).

Phentermine

Phentermine (Fastin) is a sympathomimetic anorexogenic agent. A 1968 study is the only longer-term, controlled trial of phentermine (26). In this study, 64 patients completed 36 weeks of placebo, phentermine, or placebo and phentermine on alternating days. Both phentermine groups lost approximately 13% of their initial weight, whereas the placebo group lost only 5%. Phentermine's main side effects are related to its sympathomimetic properties and include insomnia, constipation, and dry mouth. Phentermine and other sympathomimetics, such as diethylpropion and phendimetrazine, have not been studied for long-term safety and efficacy, and their use beyond 3 months is "off-label."

Medications in Clinical Trials

Several medications approved for the treatment of other conditions are sometimes used to treat obesity as well. The medications described below are currently being evaluated as antiobesity agents in phase III trials.

Bupropion (Wellbutrin)

Bupropion is an atypical antidepressant that has anecdotally been found to induce weight loss. Although the mean weight loss seen with bupropion is small, as an antidepressant it is preferable to the many drugs that may induce weight gain.

Anderson et al (27) conducted a 48-week randomized placebo-controlled trial of the weight loss effects of bupropion that compared it with a placebo, 300 mg, and 400 mg of bupropion sustained release. Percentage weight losses for subjects completing 24 weeks were 5.0%, 7.2%, and 10.1% for placebo, bupropion sustained release 300, and 400 mg/day, respectively. Bupropion is contraindicated in patients with seizures. Other side effects include dry mouth, insomnia, anxiety, increased blood pressure, and nausea.

Metformin (Glucophage)

Metformin is an antihyperglycemic agent that acts by decreasing production of glucose by the liver and increases sensitivity to insulin. Gokcel et al demonstrated that metformin achieved weight loss similar to orlistat during a 6-month period (7). Kay et al studied the effects of metformin on obese, hyperinsulinemic, nondiabetic subjects (28). When compared with placebo, the metformin group achieved significantly greater weight loss (6.5% $\pm$ 0.8% vs 3.8% $\pm$ 0.4%, $P < .01$) and improvement in their hyperinsulinemia. In patients with fasting hyperglycemia, metformin produced greater weight loss than placebo, but less than lifestyle changes alone. The average weight loss was 0.1, 2.1, and 5.6 kg in the placebo, metformin, and lifestyle-intervention groups, respectively ($P < .001$) (29).

On the basis of this evidence, metformin should be the first-line drug in obese diabetic patients. The most common side effects of metformin are nausea, flatulence, diarrhea, and bloating. The most serious side effect is lactic acidosis, but this is rare (< 1/100,000).

Topiramate (Topamax)

Topiramate is an antiepileptic agent that has been found to reduce body weight in patients with a variety of disorders, including epilepsy, bipolar disorder, and binge eating disorder (30). Randomized-controlled studies are necessary to establish the true efficacy of this medication in the treatment of obesity. At present, topiramate has been useful "off-label" for the treatment of migraine headaches and neuropathic pain; it also causes weight loss rather than the weight gain usually seen with other antiepileptics. Topiramate can cause paresthesias, cognitive side effects, as well as renal stones and, rarely, acute-angle glaucoma.

Medications in Early Development

Two medications—Axokine and Rimonabant—have been developed specifically for obesity treatment and are early in their evaluation.

Axokine

Axokine, an analog of ciliary neutrophic factor, activates leptin-like pathways, thereby reducing food intake. The phase II trials were very promising. The drug is currently in phase III trials. In a placebo-controlled study (unpublished) of 1,968 people, participants who received Axokine lost significantly more weight than placebo (6.2 vs 2.6 lb, $P < .001$)

Rimonabant

Rimonabant is a cannabinoid receptor antagonist that has shown promise in phase II trials and is now in phase III trials. It reduces hunger by blocking the cannabinoid receptors.

Medication-Induced Obesity

The role of medications as a factor that can induce weight gain is often overlooked. Some commonly prescribed medications are associated with significant weight gain. The list includes medications used to treat diabetes, depression, schizophrenia, and hypertension. When evaluating an obese patient for the first time, the clinician should do a thorough review of all current prescription and over-the-counter medications, to look for weight-gaining medications and to consider alternatives.

Conclusion

The obesity epidemic continues to grow at an alarming rate. Pharmacotherapy has been proven effective in weight reduction and in improvement of co-morbid conditions. As our understanding of obesity grows, so, too, will our armamentarium to combat this disease. There are several promising medications currently in clinical trials that induce weight loss through several separate mechanisms. Ultimately, obesity will likely be treated with combinations of medications, similar to other chronic diseases such as heart failure, hypertension, and diabetes.

References

1. Flegal KM, Carroll MD, Ogden CL, Johnson CL. Prevalence and trends in obesity among US adults, 1999–2000. *JAMA*. 2002;288:1723–1727.
2. National Institutes of Health, National Heart, Lung, and Blood Institute. *The Practical Guide: Identification, Evaluation, and Treatment of Overweight and Obesity in Adults*. Bethesda, Md: National Institutes of Health; 2002. NIH Publication No. 00-4084.
3. Bray GA, Blackburn GL, Ferguson JM, Greenway FL, Jain AK, Mendel CM, Mendels J, Ryan DH, Schwartz SL, Scheinbaum ML, Seaton TB. Sibutramine produces dose-related weight loss. *Obes Res*. 1999;7:189–198.
4. Wirth A, Krause J. Long-term weight loss with sibutramine: a randomized controlled trial. *JAMA*. 2001;286:1331–1339.
5. Apfelbaum M, Vague P, Ziegler O, Hanotin C, Thomas F, Leutenegger E. Long-term maintenance of weight loss after a very-low-calorie diet: a randomized blinded trial of the efficacy and tolerability of sibutramine. *Am J Med*. 1999;106:179–184.
6. Cueller GE, Ruiz AM, Monsalve MC. Six-month treatment of obesity with sibutramine 15 mg: a double-blind, placebo-controlled monocenter clinical trial in a Hispanic population. *Obes Res*. 2000;8:71–82.
7. Gokcel A, Gumurdulu Y, Karakose H, Melek Ertorer E, Tanaci N, Bascil-Tutuncu N, Guvener N. Evaluation of the safety and efficacy of sibutramine, orlistat and metformin in the treatment of obesity. *Diabetes Obes Metab*. 2002;4:49–55.
8. McMahon FG, Weinstein SP, Rowe E, Ernst KR, Johnson F, Fujioka K. Sibutramine is safe and effective for weight loss in obese patients whose hypertension is well controlled with angiotensin-converting enzyme inhibitors. *J Hum Hypertens*. 2002;16:5–11.

9. McMahon FG, Fujioka K, Singh BN, Mendel CM, Rowe E, Rolston K, Johnson F, Mooradian AD. Efficacy and safety of sibutramine in obese white and African American patients with hypertension: a 1-year, double-blind, placebo-controlled, multicenter trial. *Arch Intern Med.* 2000;160:2185–2191.

10. Rossner S, Sjostrom L, Noack R, Meinders AE, Noseda G. Weight loss, weight maintenance, and improved cardiovascular risk factors after 2 years treatment with orlistat for obesity. European Orlistat Obesity Study Group. *Obes Res.* 2000;8:49–61.

11. Sjostrom L, Rissanen A, Andersen T, Boldrin M, Golay A, Koppeschaar HP, Krempf M. Randomised placebo-controlled trial of orlistat for weight loss and prevention of weight regain in obese patients. European Multicentre Orlistat Study Group. *Lancet.* 1998;352:167–172.

12. Davidson MH, Hauptman J, DiGirolamo M, Foreyt JP, Halsted CH, Heber D, Heimburger DC, Lucas CP, Robbins DC, Chung J, Heymsfield SB. Weight control and risk factor reduction in obese subjects treated for 2 years with orlistat: a randomized controlled trial. *JAMA.* 1999;281:235–242.

13. Finer N, James WP, Kopelman PG, Lean ME, Williams G. One-year treatment of obesity: a randomized double-blind, placebo-controlled, multicentre study of orlistat, a gastrointestinal lipase inhibitor. *Int J Obes Relat Metab Disord.* 2000;24:306–313.

14. Hauptman J, Lucas C, Boldrin MN, Collins H, Segal KR. Orlistat in the long-term treatment of obesity in primary care settings. *Arch Fam Med.* 2000;9: 160–167.

15. Hollander PA, Elbein SC, Hirsch IB, Kelley D, McGill J, Taylor T, Weiss SR, Crockett SE, Kaplan RA, Comstock J, Lucas CP, Lodewick PA, Canovatchel W, Chung J, Hauptman J. Role of orlistat in the treatment of obese patients with type 2 diabetes. A 1-year randomized double-blind study. *Diabetes Care.* 1998;21:1288–1294.

16. Lindgarde F. The effect of orlistat on body weight and coronary heart disease risk profile in obese patients: the Swedish Multimorbidity Study. *J Intern Med.* 2000;248:245–254.

17. Kelley DE, Bray GA, Pi-Sunyer FX, Klein S, Hill J, Miles J, Hollander P. Clinical efficacy of orlistat therapy in overweight and obese patients with insulin-treated type 2 diabetes: a 1-year randomized controlled trial. *Diabetes Care.* 2002;25:1033–1041.

18. James WP, Astrup A, Finer N, Hilsted J, Kopelman P, Rossner S, Saris WH, Van Gaal LF. Effect of sibutramine on weight maintenance after weight loss: a randomised trial STORM Study Group. Sibutramine Trial of Obesity Reduction and Maintenance. *Lancet.* 2000;356:2119–2125.

19. Sramek JJ, Leibowitz MT, Weinstein SP, Rowe ED, Mendel CM, Levy B, McMahon FG, Mullican WS, Toth PD, Cutler NR. Efficacy and safety of sibutramine for weight loss in obese patients with hypertension well controlled by beta-adrenergic blocking agents: a placebo-controlled, double-blind, randomised trial. *J Hum Hypertens.* 2002;16:13–19.

20. Fujioka K, Seaton TB, Rowe E, Jelinek CA, Raskin P, Lebovitz HE, Weinstein SP. Weight loss with sibutramine improves glycaemic control and other metabolic parameters in obese patients with type 2 diabetes mellitus. *Diabetes Obes Metab.* 2000;2:175–187.

21. Zannad F, Gille B, Grentzinger A, Bruntz JF, Hammadi M, Boivin JM, Hanotin C, Igau B, Drouin P. Effects of sibutramine on ventricular dimensions and heart valves in obese patients during weight reduction. *Am Heart J.* 2002; 144:508–515.

22. Zhi J, Melia AT, Guerciolini R, Chung J, Kinberg J, Hauptman JB, Patel IH. Retrospective population-based analysis of the dose-response (fecal fat excretion) relationship of orlistat in normal and obese volunteers. *Clin Pharmacol Ther.* 1994;56:82–85.

23. Carriere F, Renou C, Ransac S, Lopez V, De Caro J, Ferrato F, De Caro A, Fleury A, Sanwald-Ducray P, Lengsfeld H, Beglinger C, Hadvary P, Verger R, Laugier R. Inhibition of gastrointestinal lipolysis by Orlistat during digestion of test meals in healthy volunteers. *Am J Physiol Gastrointest Liver Physiol.* 2001;281:G16–G28.

24. Muls E, Kolanowski J, Scheen A, VanGaal L. The effects of orlistat on weight and on serum lipids in obese patients with hypercholesterolemia: a randomized, double-blind placebo-controlled multicentre study. *Int J Obes Relat Metab Disord.* 2001;25:1713–1721.

25. Cavaliere H, Floriano I, Medeiros-Neto G. Gastrointestinal side effects of orlistat may be prevented by concomitant prescription of natural fibers (psyllium mucilloid). *Int J Obes Relat Metab Disord.* 2001;25:1095–1099.

26. Munro JF, MacCuish AC, Wilson EM, Duncan LJP. Comparison of continuous and intermittent anorectic therapy in obesity. *BMJ.* 1968;10:352–354.

27. Anderson JW, Greenway FL, Fujioka K, Gadde KM, McKenney J, O'Neil PM. Buproprion SR enhances weight loss: a 48-week double-blind, placebo-controlled trial. *Obes Res.* 2002:10:633–641.

28. Kay JP, Alemzadeh R, Langley G, D'Angelo L, Smith P, Holshouser S. Beneficial effects of metformin in normoglycemic morbidly obese adolescents. *Metabolism.* 2001;50:1457–1461.

29. Knowler WC, Barrett-Connor E, Fowler SE, Hamman RF, Lachin JM, Walker EA, Nathan DM. Reduction in the incidence of type 2 diabetes with lifestyle intervention or metformin. *N Engl J Med.* 2002;346:393–403.

30. Appolinario JC, Fontenelle LF, Papelbaum M, Bueno JR, Coutinho W. Topiramate use in obese patients with binge eating disorder: an open study. *Can J Psychiatry.* 2002;47:271–273.

PART B. Practical Applications

Cathy A. Nonas, MS, RD, CDE

Until recently, medications for the treatment of obesity were prescribed for short-term use (1). These anorexigenic medications, mostly amphetamines that increased the neurotransmitter norepinephrine, were prescribed to help patients break the cycle of overeating, with the expectation that they would then continue to lose weight on their own. This, however, was not the case. Short-term medication use was ineffective for long-term weight loss (2). More importantly, there were significant negative side effects of these anorexigenic agents, such as cardiac arrhythmias, hypertension, abuse potential, and death.

In 1992, Weintraub (3) studied a combination of two appetite suppressants—fenfluramine and phentermine. This was the first time that a medication for weight loss was studied for long-term efficacy. Although fenfluramine was later withdrawn from the market because of its side effects, its successful long-term efficacy began a new way of thinking about obesity treatment: weight-loss medication might be needed for long-term maintenance of weight loss the same way that a statin might be used for long-term lowering of lipids.

The history of weight-loss drugs, including the medications currently approved by the Food and Drug Administration (FDA), is described in this chapter, along with the differences between "cocktails" and responsible pharmacotherapy.

Case Study. Lucy—Part One

Lucy is a 57-year-old woman, 65 inches, 230 lb, body mass index (BMI) of 38, with a long history of medication use for weight loss. In 1965, at age 18 years, she was prescribed thyroid medication for weight loss, not hypothyroidism. Lucy also self-prescribed: she thought that if some thyroid medication was good, more must be better. After she was admitted to the emergency room with a cardiac arrhythmia that was due to a medication-induced thyrotoxicosis, she had to stop taking all thyroid medication.

Then Lucy turned to amphetamines to lose weight. Never fully understanding their abuse potential, Lucy took amphetamines long enough to become addicted, using them to stay awake, and another drug (valium) to help her sleep.

When Lucy was no longer getting the weight-loss effect she wanted from the amphetamines, she turned to a mixture of drugs prescribed by a weight loss "specialist." He prescribed what was called "rainbow pills," a mixture of amphetamines, thyroid, and digitalis. Digitalis was another drug used in the late 1950s and 1960s for weight loss. It is still prescribed today for heart failure, but side effects include an irregular heartbeat and loss of appetite, among other things. The rainbow mixture, very popular in the 1960s, was the cause of a number of deaths. In 1968, this combination of drugs was banned (4). When Lucy could no longer get this combination, she stopped taking all medication and promptly regained the weight she had lost, plus another 20 lb. To this day, she blames the pills for her current weight and is sure that her metabolism is "ruined," although she has never had it tested. At the same time, she feels desperate to lose weight. She is considering asking her physician for some new weight-loss medication.

Rationale for Drug Treatment of Obesity

Currently there are a number of drugs that are FDA-approved for weight-loss use, although only two are approved for long-term use. As stated in this chapter's overview section, orlistat (Xenical) and sibutramine (Meridia) produce more weight loss than dietary restriction alone, and better maintenance after weight loss (5). Why is it important to consider drugs for weight loss if their effect is minimal? The importance of this is crucial to understand.

As BMI increases, morbidity increases (6,7). Conversely, as someone loses even a little bit of weight, the health profile improves. Such improvement becomes clinically significant with 5% to 10% weight loss (8,9).

In general, studies of weight loss using regular-food diets and/or behavioral treatment report small losses and subsequent weight regain (10). Very–low-calorie diets show greater weight losses, but long-term efficacy is not much different from standard approaches (11). Maintenance data after bariatric surgery show more success, but the procedure is only available for people with BMIs of ≥40 or of ≥35 with comorbidities (see Chapter 8: Surgical Treatment). Studies of orlistat and sibutramine show greater weight losses than restricting food alone, as well as improved maintenance of weight loss (12). These studies were the foundation upon which the FDA determined that the medications should be used long-term.

Using the diabetes paradigm for comparison, medication is warranted if the patient is unable to normalize the serum glucose levels using diet and activity alone. Even with medication, the best serum glucose effect occurs when the patient can control the environment as well. If medication is withdrawn, the blood sugar may rise again, particularly at times when environmental promoters are not well controlled. It is the same with obesity. If the obese person's lifestyle does not change enough to result in weight loss—and subsequent maintenance—then medication may be warranted to help. Likewise, if an effective medication for obesity is withdrawn, weight—like blood sugar—will rise. One big difference is the number of medications that are available and have been clinically tested: if one diabetes medication is ineffective, there are many more to try. In obesity, there are only two medications currently approved for long-term use. Obese patients would benefit from more medications. Although some obesity agents are currently in development, their efficacy and potential availability is still unknown.

How Medications for Weight Loss Work

Medications approved by the FDA for weight loss can be divided by their mechanism of action: those that work centrally by affecting neurotransmission in the brain and those that act peripherally by reducing nutrient absorption in the gut. To understand the centrally acting medications, it is helpful to refer to basic physiology.

How a Neuron Works

A neuron's physiology is like a tree. Branched extensions called dendrites receive messages while a long trunk, called an axon, emits them. Messages are transmitted along the axon by an electrical impulse or action potential. When an action potential reaches the axon terminal (the transmitting end of the cell), vesicles in the terminal area release neurotransmitters (chemical agents) that can cross the tiny gap (synapse) between one neuron and another to relay the message. The neurotransmitters then attach to specific receptors on the receiving neuron, which picks up the message and, repeating the process, sends it in the form of an action potential to the next terminal.

Appetite suppressants work by increasing the availability of the monoamine neurotransmitters norepinephrine, serotonin, and, to a lesser degree, dopamine, in the central nervous system (CNS). Billions of messages are transmitted, sometimes traveling long distances from the brain down the spinal cord to peripheral nerve bodies, muscle cells, and other organs throughout the body.

When norepinephrine and serotonin are released, they exert an influence on functions throughout the body, such as arterial blood pressure, body temperature, gastrointestinal motility, and appetite, as well as neurobiological ones, such as appetite and depression (13). As clinicians, we must understand the potential side effects, to ensure that the patient is well monitored.

Selectivity

Many medications affect neurotransmission. Antidepressants are the best known. Neurotransmitters and their receptors are function specific. Prozac, for example, can reduce depression; Meridia, which affects the same neurotransmitters, can reduce appetite. The differences between the medications are attributable to their selectivity. Medications may affect reuptake of the neurotransmitter or promote its degradation, such as the enzyme monoamine oxidase, which acts to break down monoamines (14,15).

Noradrenergic Agents

For the purpose of this chapter, medication side effects can be categorized by neurotransmitter. For example, sympathomimetic noradrenergic agents (medications that affect more norepinephrine), such as phentermine, amphetamines, or diethylproprion, may cause hypertension, palpitations, insomnia, headache, dry mouth, constipation, or diarrhea (16). Two other sympathomimetic drugs are phenylpropanolamine (PPA) and ephedrine. PPA (Tavist D and Acutrim) has been removed from the market because of its adverse side effects, including its ability to increase cardiac output, which results in more strain on the heart's circulation. Ephedrine (eg, Ma Huang and ephedra) increases metabolism and stimulates cardiac output and peripheral resistance. Ephedrine, which can be bought over-the-counter, has not been approved for weight loss and has been banned in the US military and some states. Owing to its cardiovascular effects, it is also unsafe and has resulted in a number of deaths (1).

Serotonergic Agents

Serotonergic medications are best known for their effect on depression. Side effects include drowsiness, dizziness, reduced libido, and weight gain. Those medications that are less selective, such as tricyclics (eg, Elavil and Tofranil), or monoamine oxidase inhibitors (MAOIs), such as Nardil and Parnate, exhibit a side-effect profile that includes all the above symptoms, as well as noradrenergic symptoms. MAOIs have additional side effects from tyramine intake, an amino acid that is prevalent in foods such as aged cheese and wine. Side effects can include severe headaches and potentially lethal hypertension (4). Selective serotonin reuptake inhibitors (SSRIs), such as fluoxetine and sertraline, are more selective, attaching only to specific receptors. They act by delaying the reuptake of the neurotransmitter by the host neuron, keeping serotonin in the synaptic gap so that it is available longer.

Most antidepressants are known to be weight promoting. These include the medications mentioned above, as well as antiepileptic drugs such as divalproex sodium (Depakote) and gabapentin (Neurontin), and antipsychotic drugs such as chlorpromazine (Thorazine), clozapine (Clozaril), and lithium (see Box 7B.1). When a patient attempts weight loss while on these medications, weight loss may be slower and more difficult (17).

Box 7B.1. Examples of Drugs That May Promote Weight Gain

Tricyclics
Elavil
Tofranil

Lithium

Monoamine oxidase inhibitors
Nardil
Parnate

Antiepileptics
Neurontin
Depakote

Antipsychotics
Thorazine
Clozaril
Resperidal
Zyprexa

Serotonin-reuptake inhibitors
Prozac
Effexor
Zoloft

Steroid hormones
Hormonal contraceptives
Corticosteroids
Progestational steroids

Diabetes treatments
Sulfonylureas
Thiazolidinedione
Insulin

B-Adrenergic blockers

Antihistamines

Case Study. Lucy—Part Two

In 1996, Lucy tried medication for weight loss again, this time taking phentermine and fenfluramine (phen/fen). It was very effective for weight loss, and during the time she was taking it she lost 40 lb. Fenfluramine (Pondimin) and its dextroisomer, dexfenfluramine (Redux), acted both as a serotonin reuptake inhibitor and a releaser of more serotonin into the system. It was thought that this increased release of serotonin caused the dangerous disease of the heart valves (valvulopathy) seen in some patients and, ultimately, was the reason this medication was taken off the market (18). Lucy's echocardiography showed no evidence of valvulopathy. When Lucy was told to stop fenfluramine, she tried phentermine alone. Available since the 1960s, phentermine was off-patent and therefore inexpensive, and it had shown good efficacy as a single drug (19). Phentermine is approved by the FDA for short-term weight loss. Termed a "non-amphetamine amphetamine," its abuse potential is low, and Lucy's physician felt he could extend the 12-week time frame if the drug was effective in producing weight loss for Lucy. However, it was not effective. Although Lucy did not regain weight as quickly, it did not help her to lose weight either. Therefore, once again, Lucy stopped taking any medication for weight loss. And once again, she regained all her lost weight and more.

Scheduling Drugs

Scheduling is a classification the FDA imposes on the basis of potential for abuse. Schedule I and II drugs have a much higher potential for abuse. Amphetamine is Schedule II. Diethylproprion, phentermine, sibutramine, and orlistat have lower abuse potentials and are Schedule IV, which makes them a safer alternative for patients (see Table 7B.1). As already stated, sibutramine and orlistat are the only two weight-loss medications approved by the FDA for long-term use. FDA approval is based on the number of responders (those who lose > 5% weight compared with those on placebo) and the amount of average weight lost compared to those on placebo. Long-term approval is based on the number of years the medication has been studied. Indications for treatment of obesity include a BMI of ≥30 or of ≥27 with comorbid conditions.

Case Study. Lucy—Part Three

Lucy is now ready to try the latest FDA-approved weight-loss medications. She is a good candidate for them, and her physician prescribes 10 mg of Meridia, which is both a norepinephrine- and a serotonin-reuptake inhibitor. Her BMI is 35. Her medication also includes a low

Table 7B.1. Pharmacotherapy Options for Weight Loss

Generic Name	Brand Name	FDA-Approved Period for Usage	DEA Schedule
Noradrenergic agents			
Benzphetamine	Didrex	Few weeks	III
Diethylproprion	Tenuate	Few weeks	IV
Phentermine	Adipex-P	Few weeks	IV
	Fastin		
	Ionamin (slow release)		
Mazindol	Sanorex	Few weeks	IV
Serotonergic/noradrenergic agents			
Sibutamine	Meridia	Long-term	IV
Lipase inhibitor agents			
Orlistat	Xenical	Long-term	IV

dose of Wellbutrin for depression, which her primary care physician prescribed. Lucy is also taking metformin, for polycystic ovary syndrome (20). Her blood pressure is 130/85; her labs show an elevated LDL-C of 135 mg/dL and an HDL-C of 42 mg/dL, plus a triglyceride of 175 mg/dL—all indicative of metabolic syndrome. Weight loss via Meridia will result in positive effects on glycemic control, lipids, and blood pressure (21–24).

Meridia

Sibutramine (Meridia) affects food intake and is FDA approved for long-term weight management. Originally designed as an antidepressant, it was found to reduce appetite rather than depression.

Meridia is a norepinephrine-, serotonin-, and dopamine-reuptake inhibitor, with its main effects on norepinephrine followed by serotonin. It does not stimulate neurotransmitter release and has no incidence of valvular heart disease. Its safety profile is good, although there has been some concern about increases in blood pressure while taking Meridia. The use of Meridia is associated with small but clinically insignificant increases of less than 1 to 3 mm Hg for diastolic blood pressure, as well as an average increase in heart rate of approximately 4 to 5 beats per minute (24). In a small minority of patients, blood pressure and heart rate show greater increases, but the weight loss associated with Meridia can lower blood pressure as well (25). As with any medication that affects noradrenergic receptors, it is important to monitor blood pressure. Although there was some concern that Meridia would have a severe cardiovascular effect similar to that of fenfluramine, 8 years after its release there have been no cases of pulmonary hypertension or valvulopathy (26).

Meridia is prescribed in 5-, 10-, and 15-mg doses, but the standard dose is 10 mg. It has a pharmacological peak of 3 to 4 hours with food, and although generally taken once per day in the morning, it may be useful to consider prescribing Meridia according to its pharmacological peak and the patient's risk of overeating. For example, the person who tends to overeat at night might take the medication at 3 PM. As with all medication, Meridia works best when prescribed in conjunction with behavior modification.

Case Study. Lucy—Part Four

The first time the clinician meets Lucy is when she comes for behavioral/nutrition guidance after taking Meridia for 1 month. She is disappointed with her weight loss of only 4 lb. She had been hoping for magic—that her hunger would disappear, that food would become uninteresting and therefore easier to restrict, and that her weight loss would be substantial. On her first visit, she is not certain that Meridia is even working or whether her hard work is paying off. She thinks she needs the higher dose.

Most clinicians would be skeptical about Lucy trying weight-loss medication, partly because of her extensive history of medication use and partly because of the fact that nothing so far has worked to maintain her weight losses. But other facts are more persuasive: (1) Lucy is obese and the risks from the obesity are greater than the side effects of the FDA-approved medications; (2) Lucy is beginning to exhibit significant risks for diseases associated with obesity; (3) she has tried other avenues for weight loss, such as Weight Watcher's, SlimFast, Optifast, other medications, and a nutritionist; and (4) she is trying once more to improve her behavioral skills (in addition to taking Meridia), to increase her chances of success. In such a situation, if the Meridia can help her lose some weight and maintain the loss, then it is an appropriate treatment strategy.

Addressing Lucy's concern about her slow weight loss, the clinician should communicate that losing 4 lb in 1 month is considered successful, as is losing 5% to 10% of baseline weight in 6 months (27). Although research shows that higher Meridia dosages produce greater weight losses (28), there is no research to prove that increasing the dosage after some time will significantly increase the rate of weight loss. Lucy denies any side effects other than dry mouth and some constipation.

Lucy's plan:

- Return to her primary care physician for blood pressure evaluation.
- Instead of taking Meridia in the morning, Lucy will take it closer to the time when she overeats the most (Meridia has a peak action of 3 to 7 hours, depending on food intake, so it might be more effective if taken at lunch if evening presents as the highest risk for overeating.).
- Discuss increasing Meridia dose to 15 mg with her physician.
- Make necessary adjustments to diet, such as increasing fiber and recording food intake more regularly.
- Start to walk at lunch hour.
- Make appointment for follow-up visit.

Six months later, when Lucy returns for a third visit, she has lost 15 lb, which is 7% of her weight. The clinician applauds her and reminds her of the Diabetes Prevention Program data (8). She not only refuses to think this weight loss is good, but she states that she is doubly frustrated because she has not lost weight for the last month. Explaining that weight loss plateaus are normal after 6 months does not make Lucy feel better, even though she admits that this is the first time she has actually maintained any weight loss at all. She is concerned that discussing maintenance when she has lost so little weight is a sign of failure, not success.

Practitioner's Note: The patient wants to lose all the excess weight before maintaining any weight loss, and yet, rarely does. This presents a conundrum: what is the criterion for success? Is it the same for the patient and the practitioner? Has anyone broached the subject before the plateau has occurred? Does the patient have any experience with maintenance or does she only know how to lose and how to regain?

Lucy has remained on 10 mg Meridia for the entire 6 months, but once again brings up the issue of increasing the dosage. She also asks about adding Xenical. There is only one study that looks at the effect of adding Xenical vs placebo to Meridia after initial weight loss, and there was no difference (29).

Lucy's new plan:

- Return to her physician to discuss 15 mg Meridia for 1 month and then evaluate results.
- Make discussed adjustments on food records.
- Continue physical activity.
- Number 1 goal: no regain.
- Number 2 goal: weight loss.
- Reassess diet in 3 months.

The practitioner is surprised that, when Lucy returns in 3 months, she has discontinued the Meridia on her own but is now feeling desperate. Furthermore, Lucy now realizes that Meridia did have an impact, particularly since she has regained everything that she had lost with Meridia. In the interim, she went to another physician (she was ashamed to see her original physician), who prescribed a combination of tenuate, lasix, and potassium. She lost a little weight with this but was concerned that this combination was not appropriate, and she did not feel comfortable with this new physician. Finally, she swallowed her pride and returned to her own primary care physician, who prescribed Xenical with the caveat that she return to a practitioner who could help her with lifestyle changes.

Xenical

Unlike other FDA-approved weight-loss medications, orlistat (Xenical) is the first nonsystemic weight-loss medication, acting entirely on the gut, not the brain. Weight loss occurs because of reduced absorption of fat calories. Triglycerides are digested by lipase enzymes into monocylglycerols and free fatty acids. These structures attach to bile salt molecules and phospholipids, forming an aggregate called a micelle. The micelles enable the fat to be absorbed into the intestinal epithelium. Xenical forms a covalent bond with some of the gastric and pancreatic lipase, essentially blocking its ability to break down fat and causing about 30% of dietary fat to be eliminated in the stool. Approved in 1999 for long-term use, Xenical has been evaluated extensively and has a strong safety record (30).

Xenical is to be taken three times per day, at meals. Since its mechanism of action is influenced by the amount of fat in the meal, when someone is following a low-fat diet, side effects are few; however, when someone consumes a lot of fat, side effects can be great, including oily stools, severe diarrhea, and stomach cramping.

Case Study. Lucy—Conclusion

Lucy is hesitant about trying Xenical. She is nervous about the side effects and states that she follows a low-fat diet, rendering the medication unnecessary.

Practitioner's Note: This is a common conflict for patients: they are nervous about the side effects and yet feel that the medication will not work because there is so little fat in the diet. In fact, Xenical is prescribed in conjunction with a low-fat diet to avoid undue side effects. It also acts as a deterrent to overindulgence in fatty foods; and the medication blocks absorption of one third of the fat that is consumed, no matter how much fat is consumed. Therefore, on a maintenance diet of 2,000 kcal, where 30% of total calories is fat, the use of Xenical will still result in a net elimination of about 200 kcal per day.

Lucy's fears can be addressed by the suggestion that she take a *teaspoon* of soluble fiber at breakfast and dinner, to reduce any side effects that may occur from any surprisingly high-fat meal she may consume (31).

After her conversation with the practitioner, Lucy is ready to try Xenical. They discuss a multivitamin to be taken either before bed or 2 hours before or after Xenical has been taken. Although no vitamin deficiencies have been seen, because of its ability to block absorption of dietary fat, Xenical has been shown to decrease the uptake of some fat-soluble vitamins and beta carotene (32).

The first week Lucy loses 2.5 lb. Mainly because she was so afraid of the side effects, she barely eats at all. By the end of the 6th week, she's testing the medication to see whether she will get side effects. By the end of the 3rd month, she has lost 10 lb, but she is finding she can eat more. By the 6th month, she has adapted well enough to Xenical so that she has lost 13 lb. Lucy is now fighting the same issues she was fighting with Meridia (which gave her similar weight losses)—she wants magic, but realistically understands that that is not a viable solution. The clinician suggests that she exercise more and do food records more consistently. But the clinician also points out how successful she has been. Her latest labs show a decrease in her LDL-C, serum triglycerides, and blood pressure (33–35). Nevertheless, she is disheartened. Lucy understands the scientific criteria for success, but she has greater expectations and she is getting tired. Together, Lucy and her clinician decide that she will try to maintain her 13 lb for a while (which, the clinician tells her, is difficult enough) and that when she is ready to restrict more, they will work together on a plan. Meanwhile, she should continue with the weight-loss medication.

Final Note

Medications for weight loss have had a dubious history, because of inappropriate practices and short-term effects. However, the newest medications (orlistat and sibutramine) have been on the market for 5 and 8 years, respectively, and their safety profiles remain good. Unfortunately, the public has high expectations. Medication is not magic. The hard work of lifestyle change still has to be done. These facts must be communicated to patients, and it should be emphasized that these medications result in greater weight loss than restricting food alone. Because weight loss means an improved health profile, medications that have a good safety record and provide weight-loss efficacy should be strongly considered for appropriate patients.

References

1. Yanovski SZ, Yanovski JA. Obesity. *N Engl J Med*. 2002;346:591–602.
2. Fujioka K. Management of obesity as a chronic disease: nonpharmacologic, pharmacologic, and surgical options. *Obes Res*. 2002;10(Suppl):116S–123S.
3. Weintraub M. Long-term weight control: the National Heart, Lung, and Blood Institute funded multimodal intervention study. *Clin Pharmacol Ther*. 1992;51:581–646.
4. Kramer, PD. *Listening to Prozac*. New York, NY: Viking; 1993.
5. Glazer G. Long-term pharmacotherapy of obesity 2000: a review of efficacy and safety. *Arch Intern Med*. 2001;161:1814–1822.
6. Institutes of Medicine. *Weighing the Options: Criteria for Evaluating Weight-Management Programs*. Washington, DC: National Academy Press; 1995.
7. World Health Organization. *Preventing and Managing the Global Epidemic: Report of a WHO Consultation on Obesity*. Geneva, Switzerland: World Health Organization; 1998.
8. Knowler WC, Barrett-Connor E, Fowler SE, Hamman RF, Lachin JM, Walker EA, Nathan DM. Reduction in the incidence of type 2 diabetes with lifestyle intervention or metformin. *N Engl J Med*. 2002;346:393–403.
9. Aronne LJ. Modern medical management of obesity: the role of pharmaceutical intervention. *J Am Diet Assoc*. 1998;98(10 Suppl 2):S23–S26.
10. Nonas C. A model of chronic care of obesity through dietary treatment. *J Am Diet Assoc*. 1998;98:S16–S22.
11. Saris WH. Very-low-calorie diets and sustained weight loss. *Obes Res*. 2001; 9(Suppl 4):295S–301S.

12. Haddock CK, Poston WSC, Dill PL, Foreyt JP, Ericsson M. Pharmacotherapy for obesity: a quantitative analysis of four decades of published randomized clinical trials. *Int J Obes Relat Metab Disord.* 2002;26:262–273.

13. Guyton AC. The nervous system. In: Guyton AC. *Textbook of Medical Physiology.* 7th ed. Philadelphia, Pa: WB Saunders; 1986:546–696.

14. Salzman B. *Psychiatric Drugs.* New York, NY: Henry Holt and Co; 1991.

15. Bray GA, Tartaglia LA. Medicinal strategies in the treatment of obesity. *Nature.* 2000;404:672–677.

16. Bray GA. Pharmacological treatment of obesity. In: Bray GA, Bouchard C, eds. *Handbook of Obesity.* New York, NY: Marcel Dekker; 1998:953–975.

17. Aronne LJ. Classification of obesity and assessment of obesity-related health risks. *Obes Res.* 2002;10(Suppl 2):105S–115S.

18. Gardin JM, Schumacher D, Constantine F, Davis KD, Leung C, Reid CL. Valvular abnormalities and cardiovascular status following exposure to dexfenfluramine or phentermine/fenfluramine. *JAMA.* 2000;283:1703–1709.

19. Munro JF, MacCuish AC, Wilson EM, Duncan LJP. Comparison of continuous and intermittent anorectic therapy in obesity. *BMJ.* 1968;1:352–354.

20. Ng EH, Wat NM, Ho PC. Effects of metformin on ovulation rate, hormonal and metabolic profiles in women with clomiphene-resistant polycystic ovaries: a randomized, double-blinded placebo-controlled trial. *Hum Reprod.* 2001;8: 1625–1631.

21. Gokcel A, Gumurdulu Y, Karakose H, Melek Ertorer E, Tanaci N, Bascil-Tutuncu N, Guvener N. Evaluation of the safety and efficacy of sibutramine, orlistat and metformin in the treatment of obesity. *Diabetes Obes Metab.* 2002;4:49–55.

22. Blackburn GL, Fernstrom MH. Toward optimal health: the experts discuss weight control drugs. *J Womens Health Gend Based Med.* 2001;10:101–107.

23. Finer N, Bloom SR, Frost GS, Banks LM, Griffiths J. Sibutramine is effective for weight loss and diabetic control in obesity with type 2 diabetes: a randomised, double-blind, placebo-controlled study. *Diabetes Obes Metab.* 2000; 2:105–112.

24. Sharma AM. Sibutramine in overweight/obese hypertensive patients. *Int J Obes Relat Metab Disord.* 2001;25(Suppl 4):S20–S23.

25. Pischon T, Sharma AM. Recent developments in the treatment of obesity-related hypertension. *Curr Opin Nephrol Hypertens.* 2002;5:497–502.

26. Narkiewicz K. Sibutramine and its cardiovascular profile. *Int J Obes Relat Metab Disord.* 2002;26(Suppl 4):S38–S41.

27. National Institutes of Health, National Heart, Lung, and Blood Institute. *Clinical Guidelines on the Identification, Evaluation, and Treatment of Overweight and Obesity in Adults.* Bethesda, Md: National Institutes of Health; 2002. NIH Publication No. 00-4084.

28. Bray GA, Blackburn GL, Ferguson JM, Greenway FL, Jain AK, Mendel CM, Mendels J, Ryan DH, Schwartz SL, Scheinbaum ML, Seaton TB. Sibutramine produces dose-related weight loss. *Obes Res.* 1999;7:189–198.

29. Wadden TA, Berkowitz RI, Womble LG, Sarwer DB, Arnold ME, Steinberg CM. Effects of sibutramine plus orlistat in obese women following 1 year of treatment by sibutramine alone: a placebo-controlled trial. *Obes Res.* 2000;8: 431–437.

30. Kushner, R. Pharmacologic Therapy. In: Bessesen DH, Kushner RF, eds. *Evaluation and Management of Obesity*. Philadelphia, Pa: Hanley & Belfus Inc; 2002:97–105.

31. Cavaliere H, Floriano I, Medeiros-Neto G. Gastrointestinal side effects of orlistat may be prevented by concomitant prescription of natural fibers (psyllium muciloid). *Int J Obes Rel Metab Disord*. 2001;25:1095–1099.

32. Finer N, James WP, Kopelman PG, Lean ME, Williams G. One-year treatment of obesity: a randomized, double-blind, placebo-controlled, multicentre study of orlistat, a gastrointestinal lipase inhibitor. *Int J Obes Relat Metab Disord*. 2000;24:306–313.

33. Heymsfield SB, Segal KR, Hauptman J, Lucas CP, Boldrin MN, Rissanen A, Wilding JP, Sjostrom L. Effects of weight loss with orlistat on glucose tolerance and progression to type 2 diabetes in obese adults. *Arch Intern Med*. 2000;160:1321–1326.

34. Reaven G, Segal K, Hauptman J, Boldrin M, Lucas C. Effect of orlistat-assisted weight loss in decreasing coronary heart disease risk in patients with syndrome X. *Am J Cardiol*. 2001;87:827–831.

35. Wierzbicki AS, Reynolds TM, Crook MA. Usefulness of orlistat in the treatment of severe hypertriglyceridemia. *Am J Cardiol*. 2002;89:229–231.

Chapter 8
Surgical Treatment

PART A. Overview

Patricia S. Choban, MD

Obesity is a chronic, progressive disease with a wide spectrum of severity. Small degrees of overweight can have substantial, cumulative adverse health consequences. Individuals with the highest level of obesity (body mass index [BMI] ≥ 40) suffer premature death and extreme detrimental health effects (1). While the overall prevalence of obesity has increased significantly (see Chapter 1: Obesity: An Overview), the prevalence of extreme obesity has tripled over the last decade (2).

Extreme, or Class III, obesity describes those individuals with BMI ≥ 40, although the term "morbid obesity" remains in use because it is linked to the diagnostic codes (ICD-9) used by health care providers and third-party payers. Surgery becomes a consideration in these patients as well as those with a BMI ≥ 35 with obesity-related comorbid diseases. Obesity-related comorbid diseases are conditions that worsen as weight increases but generally improve or resolve as weight decreases. These conditions include type 2 diabetes mellitus, hypertension, hyperlipidemia, obstructive sleep apnea, urinary stress incontinence, gastroesophageal reflux disease, and joint pain—to name a few. Weight loss from gastric bypass has also been shown to reduce the risk of premature death (3). Patients who qualify for surgery but do not receive the treatment, because of personal choice, financial issues, or lack of direction from their health care providers, are at a

4.5-fold increased risk of death each year compared with those who received surgical treatment (3). Given the increasing prevalence of severe obesity and the limited long-term effectiveness of traditional means of dietary restriction, this dramatic reduction in risk of premature death underscores the need for urgent consideration of surgery in this population. It is for this reason that surgical treatment of obesity is increasingly being used worldwide. The purpose of this chapter is to review the history, procedures, and mechanisms of bariatric surgery.

The History of Bariatric Surgery: Malabsorption vs Restriction

Malabsorption

Jejunoileal bypass (also known as intestinal bypass or JIB) was the first surgical treatment for extreme obesity and was developed almost 40 years ago. JIB was much more malabsorptive than most of the surgeries used today. JIB short-circuited the small intestine, connecting the first 8 inches of jejunum to the last 12 inches of ileum. The excluded limb of the small bowel was "vented" to the colon or the small intestine, so it was not obstructed, but there were no intestinal contents passing through. The mechanism of action was malabsorptive, and JIB remains the example, albeit bad, of a purely malabsorptive operation. JIB resulted in weight loss primarily from changes in nutrient absorption. The "blind loop" of a JIB resulted in a myriad of problems, and when combined with severe nutritional and metabolic complications, led to the procedure being abandoned in the early 1980s (4,5). It was apparent that the problem of severe obesity was persistent, and other procedures were developed to address this serious condition.

Restriction

Initially, the pendulum swung toward restrictive procedures, which functioned by reductions in intake. The simplicity of purely restrictive procedures was inviting, and a number of variants developed almost simultaneously. Restrictive procedures decrease the size of the stomach by division, partitioning, or removal. The amount of stomach removed or excluded, in combination with the size of the outlet, determined the degree of restriction. With time, restrictive procedures have included gastric banding, gastric bubbles, and horizontal stapled gastroplasty. Horizontal gastroplasty earned the nickname "stomach stapling" and was an ineffective procedure because it "unzipped" in 90% of patients within 3 years of surgery. The interest in gastroplasty remained, and the procedure was eventually modified to the more durable vertical banded gastroplasty. The newest addition to this category is the adjustable silicone gastric band. These restrictive procedures work entirely by decreasing intake and creating satiety. No portion of the GI tract is bypassed. In general, restrictive procedures are technically simple, and nutritional deficiencies related to malabsorption are not an issue. The drawback has been weight regain in long-term follow-up, as well as mechanical difficulties with certain textures of food (eg, red meats and noncrumbly breads).

Restriction and Malabsorption

At about the same time JIB was introduced, Mason and Ito (6) introduced a gastric bypass procedure that, although primarily restrictive, had a malabsorptive component. The gastric bypass was initially performed as a loop but was quickly modified to a Roux-en-Y bypass (7). During the past 3 or 4 decades, this operation has remained relatively intact and is now the most common surgical procedure performed for weight loss in the United States. The combination of restriction and a small degree of malabsorption has made this surgery the most successful for long-term weight loss, with side effects that are generally manageable.

Current Practice: Anatomy and Outcomes

Although most US surgeons perform Roux-en-Y gastric bypass for the treatment of extreme obesity, procedures other than gastric bypass are also being performed. Thus, it behooves those caring for obese patients to be familiar with the four procedures currently in use (see Figure 8A.1) (8). From restrictive to malabsorptive in mechanism, the procedures are:

1. Adjustable silicone gastric banding (AGB)
2. Vertical banded gastroplasty (VBG)
3. Roux-en-Y gastric bypass (RYGB)
4. Biliopancreatic diversion (BPD), with or without duodenal switch

In general, as the degree of malabsorption increases, weight loss and the incidence of complications increase. The procedure selected for a specific patient may vary and tends to be surgeon specific. Some surgeons use the same procedure in all settings, which allows the program to gain a focused experience and predictability. Some surgeons offer different procedures and make a decision with the patient based on degree of obesity, side-effects tolerance, and perceived reliability for follow-up. This is the "art" of medicine, because there are few data to predict, on an individual basis, outcome with a specific procedure.

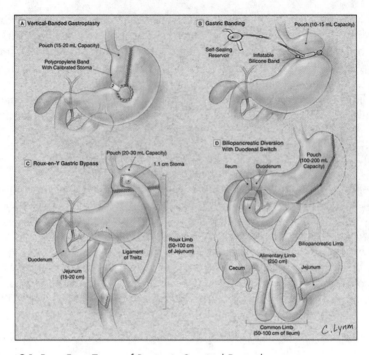

Figure 8A.1.   Four Types of Bariatric Surgical Procedures
Reprinted with permission from Brolin RE. Bariatric surgery and long-term control of morbid obesity. *JAMA.* 2002;288:2793–2796. Copyright © 2002, American Medical Association. All rights reserved.

Weight loss after surgery is generally expressed as the percent of excess weight lost. The excess is the actual weight less the ideal body weight. This number is fairly predictable for different procedures (ranging from 35% to 75% 1 to 2 years after surgery) and can help estimate expected weight loss in patients 100 lb overweight or 500 lb overweight. For example, Linda, a 66-inch woman   (ideal body weight 137 lb), who started out at 330 lb, would have 193 lb of excess weight. If she lost 135 lb, that would equal 70% of the excess weight and 41% of her actual body weight. Her 66-inch sister, Lisa, who started out at 240 lb, would have 103 lb of excess; 70% of her excess weight would be a 72-lb weight loss, and this would be 30% of her actual body weight lost.

Adjustable Gastric Banding

AGB places a silicone band around the upper stomach, just below the gastroesophageal junction. The band is connected to a port placed subcutaneously. The port is accessed percutaneously, and the size of the band is changed by injecting or removing saline. The band, which determines pouch outlet size, can be adjusted in accordance with the rate of weight loss. The device received Food and Drug Administration approval in June 2001 for use in the United States. Long-term data on American patients are not available, but preliminary data not as good as those seen in Europe and Australia (9). The AGB achieves an average weight loss of 35% to 50% of initial excess body weight (9,10), or, for Lisa, 15% in initial weight; for Linda, 20% in initial weight. The incidence and severity of complications are lower after laparoscopic adjustable gastric banding than after gastric bypass or gastroplasty (11). Unique complications include band slippage, esophageal dilatation, erosion of the band into the stomach, and band or port infections. Balloon or system leaks can diminish weight loss and require additional procedures.

Vertical Banded Gastroplasty

VBG involves constructing a 15- to 30-mL vertical gastric pouch below the gastroesophageal junction (12). This small gastric reservoir empties into the remaining stomach through an outlet that is restricted by a band. The band may be constructed of polypropylene mesh or of a ring of sialastic tubing. Weight loss averages 40% to 50% of the excess body weight. Postoperative complications that are specifically associated with gastroplasty include stomal stenosis, staple line disruption, erosion of the band, and gastroesophageal reflux.

Gastroplasty does not cause dumping syndrome, iron deficiency, or vitamin B-12 deficiency. When compared with RYGB, VBG has a lower initial weight loss and greater weight regain (13). Overall complication rate, however, is similar between the two procedures. For these reasons, RYGB has become the more prevalent procedure.

Roux-en-Y Gastric Bypass and Biliopancreatic Diversion: The "Y" Limb

Before reviewing RYGB and BPD procedures (described below), it is important to understand a key feature of both procedures—a "Y" limb. The bypass component of procedures is accomplished by creating a "Y" with the small intestine. The most proximal small bowel remains attached to the stomach and/or duodenum below the gastric division or partition. This limb can be called the pancreobiliary limb, because it drains bile and pancreatic digestive enzymes. The next limb drains the small pouch; hence, it carries only food. This is the Roux limb. The point at which the pancreobiliary limb connects into the Roux limb forms the Y. At this point, the digestive juices and food mix and proceed together, and the remaining arm of the Y is called the common channel. On average, adults have about 600 cm of small bowel. Increasing the length of one limb decreases the length of the other two limbs (Figure 8A.2).

Roux-en-Y Gastric bypass

RYGB starts with the creation of a 10- to 30-mL proximal gastric pouch by either stapling or transecting the stomach. The outlet of the pouch is anastomosed to the Roux limb. The length of bowel exposed to nutrients determines the degree of malabsorption associated with the gastric bypass. A 45- to 100-cm limb (proximal or short-limb gastric bypass) is often used in patients with a BMI of <50, whereas a limb of 150 cm or more (long-limb gastric bypass) is often used in patients with a BMI of >50 (14). Modifications that shorten the common channel (<200 cm) increase the degree of malabsorption, making the procedure more like a BPD and may be referred to as a distal gastric bypass. Gastric bypass results in weight loss of 50% to 65% of excess body weight, which corresponds to about 30% to 40% of total body weight. General complications that can occur after any intestinal operation include hemorrhage, gastrointestinal leak with peritonitis, splenic injury, and wound infection. Complications that are more specific to gastric procedures include stomal stenosis, marginal ulcers, staple line disruption, dilation of the bypassed stomach, internal hernias, specific nutrient deficiencies (iron, calcium, folic acid, and vitamin B-12), and dumping syndrome (15).

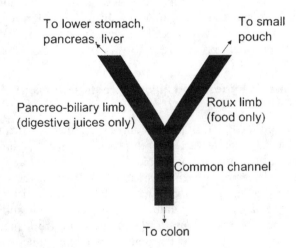

Figure 8A.2. The Y Limb

The Biliopancreatic Diversion

BPD causes significant malabsorption as well as gastric restriction. It can achieve more weight loss than that usually achieved with gastric bypass or vertical banded gastroplasty and has been advocated for use in patients with the most extreme obesity. This procedure involves resecting 60% of the stomach. The proximal duodenum is transected and anastomosed to the distal intestine, 250 cm proximal to the ileocecal valve. The distal end of the duodenum is closed, and the proximal intestine is connected to the ileum, 100 cm from the ileocecal valve. Therefore, this procedure generates a 150-cm Roux limb that connects with the stomach, and a 100-cm "common channel" that allows mixing of digestive enzymes and bile salts with ingested food. The duodenal switch modification of the procedure preserves the pylorus and the physiological function of the stomach, thereby decreasing the risk of marginal ulcers and eliminating the risk of dumping syndrome. These procedures achieve weight loss of 55% to 75% of excess body weight. They have greater risk of nutritional-deficiency states and require more frequent follow-up (16). The perioperative risks are similar to those of gastric bypass.

Laparoscopic Procedures

How the procedure is accomplished, whether "open" (with a 6- to 8-inch incision and the surgeon's hands touching the bowels) or laparoscopically (with multiple small incisions allowing ports for surgical instruments and camera placement), is less important than the actual procedure performed. The first series of patients with laparoscopic gastric bypass was reported in 1994 (17). The conversion of surgeons to the laparoscopic approach has been gradual. Laparoscopic bariatric surgery is technically demanding, and most bariatric procedures are still being done in an open fashion. Procedures that have been done laparoscopically include vertical banded gastroplasty, gastric bypass, duodenal switch, and BPD, as well as the more recent adjustable banding procedures (18). Open procedures are performed more rapidly, shortening the duration of anesthesia. Laparoscopic procedures have been associated with fewer wound problems, including hernias. As noted, the laparoscopic procedures are technically challenging and have been associated with an increased risk of leaks, especially early in a surgeon's experience.

Mechanisms

Reduced Intake

Surgical treatment for obesity results in weight loss, because energy intake is less than energy expenditure. Most of this is accomplished by early satiety and a decrease in total intake. Fat malabsorption, gastrointestinal side effects, and dumping syndrome can result in unpleasant consequences and can also modify nutrient intake. In the more malabsorptive procedures, nutrients are simply not absorbed.

Energy Expenditure

Effects of bariatric surgery on energy expenditure are not well understood. Bypassing the lower stomach and proximal small intestine appears to blunt the "starvation" response. After gastric bypass, patients maintain a resting metabolic rate within about 15% of their Harris Benedict–predicted metabolic rate, in spite of caloric restriction in the 800- to 1,000-kcal range. This effect is maintained for up to 2 years (19).

Taste, Satiety, and Hunger

Changes in taste acuity occur after gastric bypass, with some patients developing an aversion to sweets that seems unrelated to the effects of dumping (20). The factors mediating the changes in satiety, energy expenditure, and taste have not been well established. The identification of the dramatic reduction in ghrelin levels after gastric bypass has been exciting. This is in contrast with an increase in ghrelin levels in nonsurgical patients losing weight with dietary restriction alone (21). This is a fascinating addition in our attempt to understand differences in hunger mediation.

Nutritional Follow-up

Nutritional and metabolic complications are not common when patients are compliant with prescribed supplements and follow-up visits are appropriately scheduled. The incidence of sequelae is related to the procedure performed. The risk of protein calorie malnutrition (PCM) has been related to the length of the common channel. When the channel is approximately 50 cm, the incidence of PCM is about 26%; when it is 75 cm, PCM incidence is about 13% (22). When the common channel is 150 cm, the incidence of PCM is about 8%, and when it is >200 cm, the incidence is <1% (23). Patients with more distal procedures should have serum albumin levels monitored several times per year in the first 3 to 4 years and then annually. With RYGB (common channel >200 cm) and VBG, PCM occurs if there is excessive vomiting or inadequate intake.

There is a decrease in iron, folate, and vitamin B-12 absorption in all procedures that bypass the lower stomach and proximal small bowel. Because of this, all patients need to be supplemented with a multivitamin. Even with supplementation, iron and vitamin B-12 deficiency may occur. Iron deficiency may result in 20% to 50% of patients, with menstruating females being at greatest risk. Vitamin B-12 deficiency may be seen in 25% to 35% of patients and warrants monitoring and treatment as indicated (15). Fat malabsorption may be seen as the common channel length decreases. When the common channel is <150 cm, the degree of malabsorption warrants supplementation with the fat-soluble vitamins A and D on a daily basis. Iron, vitamin B-12, and complete blood count are monitored twice a year in the first 2 years and then annually.

Conclusion

Obesity surgery has become mainstream therapy for extreme obesity, which is increasing in prevalence. It is very effective in reducing weight and is currently the most effective long-term therapy for extreme obesity. The complication rate is low, and most complications are manageable, especially if diagnosed promptly.

References

1. Clinical Guidelines on the Identification, Evaluation, and Treatment of Overweight and Obesity in Adults—the evidence report. National Institutes of Health. *Obes Res*. 1998;6(Suppl 2):51S–209S.
2. Freedman DS, Khan LK, Serdula MK, Galuska DA, Dietz WH. Trends and correlates of class 3 obesity in the United States from 1990 through 2000. *JAMA*. 2002;288:1758–1761.
3. MacDonald KG Jr, Long SD, Swanson MS, Brown BM, Morris P, Dohm GL, Pories WJ. The gastric bypass operation reduces the progression and mortality of non-insulin-dependent diabetes mellitus. *J Gastrointest Surg*. 1997;1:213–220.
4. Payne JH, DeWind LT. Surgical treatment of obesity. *Am J Surg*. 1969;118:141–147.
5. Hocking MP, Duerson MC, O'Leary JP, Woodward ER. Jejunoileal bypass for morbid obesity. Late follow-up in 100 cases. *N Engl J Med*. 1983;308:995–999.
6. Mason EE, Ito CC. Gastric bypass in obesity. *Surg Clin North Am*. 1967;47:1345–1351.
7. Griffen WO Jr, Young VL, Stevenson CC. A prospective comparison of gastric and jejunoileal bypass procedures for morbid obesity. *Ann Surg*. 1977;186:500–509.
8. Brolin RE. Bariatric surgery and long-term control of morbid obesity. *JAMA*. 2002;288:2793–2796.
9. DeMaria EJ. Laparoscopic adjustable silicone gastric banding. *Surg Clin North Am*. 2001;81:1129–1144.

10. Hauri P, Steffen R, Ricklin T, Riedmann HJ, Sendi P, Horber FF. Treatment of morbid obesity with the Swedish adjustable gastric band (SAGB): complication rate during a 12-month follow-up period. *Surgery.* 2000;127:484–488.

11. Nguyen NT, Goldman C, Rosenquist CJ, Arango A, Cole CJ, Lee SJ, Wolfe BM. Laparoscopic versus open gastric bypass: a randomized study of outcomes, quality of life, and costs. *Ann Surg.* 2001;234:279–289.

12. Doherty C. Vertical banded gastroplasty. *Surg Clin North Am.* 2001;81:1097–1112.

13. Sugerman HJ, Starkey JV, Birkenhauer RA. A randomized prospective trial of gastric bypass versus vertical banded gastroplasty for morbid obesity and their effects on sweets versus non sweets eaters. *Ann Surg.* 1987;205:613–624.

14. Brolin RE, Kenler HA, Gorman RC, Cody RP. Long-limb gastric bypass in the superobese: a prospective randomized study. *Ann Surg.* 1992;215:387–395.

15. Brolin RE. Gastric bypass. *Surg Clin North Am.* 2001;81:1077–1095.

16. Marceau P, Biron S, Hould F-S, Lebel S, Marceau S. Malabsorption procedure in surgical treatment of morbid obesity. *Problems in General Surgery.* 2000; 14:29–39.

17. Wittgrove AC, Clark GW, Tremblay LJ. Laparoscopic gastric bypass, Roux-en-Y: preliminary report of five cases. *Obes Surg.* 1994;4:353–357.

18. Schauer PR, Ikramuddin S. Laparoscopic surgery for morbid obesity. *Surg Clin North Am.* 2001;81:1145–1179.

19. Flancbaum L, Choban PS, Bradley LR, Burge JC. Changes in measured resting energy expenditure after Roux-en-Y gastric bypass for clinically severe obesity. *Surgery.* 1997;122:943–949.

20. Burge JC, Schaumburg JZ, Choban PS, DiSilvestro RA, Flancbaum L. Changes in patients' taste acuity after Roux-en-Y gastric bypass for clinically severe obesity. *J Am Diet Assoc.* 1995;95:666–670.

21. Cummings DE, Weigle DS, Frayo RS, Breen PA, Ma MK, Dellinger EP, Purnell JQ. Plasma ghrelin levels after diet-induced weight loss or gastric bypass surgery. *N Engl J Med.* 2002;346:1623–1630.

22. Scopinaro N, Adami GF, Marinari GM, Gianetta E, Traverso E, Friedman D, Camerini G, Baschieri G, Simonelli A. Biliopancreatic diversion. *World J Surg.* 1998;22:936–946.

23. Sugerman HJ, Kellum JM, DeMaria EJ. Conversion of proximal to distal gastric bypass for failed gastric bypass for superobesity. *J Gastrointest Surg.* 1997;1:517–525.

PART B. Practical Applications

Allison Schimmel Mattson, MS, RD

Many clinicians have encountered patients who have either had some type of bariatric surgery, want information regarding bariatric surgery, or are candidates for bariatric surgery. Many professionals, however, are uncomfortable working with these patients because of the lack of information regarding the postoperative treatment of these individuals. In addition, most research has been done primarily by bariatric surgeons, dealing more with outcomes of different procedures than with guidelines for the long-term treatment of the bariatric surgery patient. This chapter reviews nutritional guidelines for the bariatric patient and is based on the available research and the experiences of bariatric clinicians.

Pretreatment Issues

Equipment

Before reviewing treatment issues, practitioners should note that special equipment is necessary to effectively assist bariatric surgery patients. In a hospital setting, special equipment for the operating room, office visits, and waiting rooms are essential, to effectively and compassionately treat larger individuals. In outpatient settings, special attention should be paid to the weight capacity of chairs, scales, and the distance the individual may need to walk to get to the office (see Part B of Chapter 4: Behavioral Treatment). This minimizes possible embarrassment for the individual and keeps the focus on education and counseling.

The Bariatric Team

Bariatric patients typically require a range of care that includes, but is not limited to, surgical, psychological, nutritional, and medical expertise. The best bariatric practices consist of several of these support people from a variety of disciplines. The particular members of that group may differ from institution to institution, and the roles of these individuals may also vary. It is essential, however, that patients are referred to the appropriate clinician when indicated and that preoperative and postoperative care is managed by the team.

Preoperative Assessment

Preoperative evaluation to assess significant comorbid conditions includes the standard surgical laboratory and radiographic studies. Pulmonary function tests, gallbladder ultrasonography, cardiac evaluation, and upper gastrointestinal fluoroscopy are also obtained when indicated. Specialty consults may be required before surgery, based on the individual assessment by the surgeon. Comorbidities often do not exclude patients from consideration for surgery but may change the surgical and anesthetic management of the patient in the perioperative phase.

Nutrition Education

Nutrition education is also an important element of the preoperative process. Before surgery, patients often benefit from practical information about the postoperative diet of the typical bariatric surgery patient. A good understanding of the physiological changes of gastric capacity and function, dietary restrictions, and potential nutrition problems is beneficial for a good outcome. Patients unable to understand these issues may be considered inappropriate or more "risky" for this surgery and probably necessitate more in-depth education before surgery. It is also recommended that patients be provided with written information for constant reinforcement of dietary guidelines. Some bariatric dietitians provide their patients with shopping lists, to minimize work for the patient after surgery. Recommendations for supplements and foods will be provided in the Perioperative Management section, below.

Behavior Modification

Behavior modification should also be discussed in the preoperative nutrition instructions. Even though food and portion control will be restricted, patients must also follow very specific behavior guidelines during ingestion. The list below describes the behaviors that will minimize problems associated with food intake:

- Chew food until puree in consistency.
- Sit down for meals and avoid "eating on the go."
- Minimize ingesting liquids and solids at the same time, especially soon after surgery. This usually causes excess intake and probable regurgitation. With time, some patients do learn how to incorporate eating and drinking at the same meal.
- Use caution when introducing a new food.
- Food and liquids should be ingested slowly.

- Avoid eating during stressful situations.
- Portion out meals to avoid overeating—use food models, measuring instruments, food diagrams, and so forth, to provide a visual tool.

Case Study. Jane

Jane comes to see you after having a gastric bypass procedure 3 months earlier. She is losing weight (approximately 10 lb per month), yet is having problems with her diet. She complains of vomiting after eating most foods and reports that she has the most trouble with liquids. She also reports significant stressors associated with her new job and her husband.

After reviewing the types of foods and portions Jane is consuming (see Chapter 2: Assessment), it would be helpful to discuss her specific eating behaviors. Does she eat and drink at the same time? Does she eat under stressful situations? Does she take the time to sit down and chew her food adequately? If a mechanical problem is not suspected, it is likely that her eating behaviors are causing the vomiting. It would be helpful to review the suggestions listed above and assess her current adherence to them. Patients often need to be reminded about the importance of appropriate eating behaviors.

Perioperative Management

Perioperative management focuses on minimizing possible postoperative complications. This involves standard postoperative processes, as well those specific to the obese individual. Venous access and fluid management need to be addressed. Although most patients are extubated soon after surgery, pulmonary function and gas exchange must be monitored carefully, particularly for those individuals with sleep apnea or obesity hypoventilation syndrome.

Early ambulation is critical and should be encouraged by the entire bariatric team. Immobility will increase the risk of pneumonia, blood clots, and constipation. Patients should also be aware, before surgery, that they will not be allowed to eat or drink or take oral medications until the surgical team gives permission. (It is essential that the team be aware of all the patient's medications.) Family members and friends should not bring any food or drink into the hospital room. Many surgeons also require a gastrograffin swallow radiograph before intake. The radiograph will rule out an anastomotic leak, which may require immediate reoperation if detected.

Typically, unless there is a complication, patients begin oral intake within 2 days of surgery. Fortunately, complications are minimal with the gastric bypass procedure, and oral intake can be initiated without a problem. More often than not, patients begin with small volumes of water and ice chips (approximately 1 oz). Most patients are thirsty but not hungry after surgery, so they characteristically welcome the introduction of water without concern for food intake. It is also not unusual for patients to express a fear of the initiation of food intake. It is important to assure the patient that this is a common concern and is critical to overcome while in the hospital. If a problem were to exist from oral intake, the difficulty would be investigated before discharge. Occasional regurgitation is common for bariatric surgery patients as they learn to consume smaller portions.

Progression of the diet is usually developed by the nutrition department of the institution and should be provided to the patient before surgery. It is also useful to educate the dietary staff and nurses caring for these individuals regarding the bariatric diet. This should eliminate confusion by the hospital staff and minimize possible complications from inappropriate food intake.

The guidelines in Table 8B.1 are indicated for patients without complications from surgery, although variations do exist based on the length of the hospital stay and the medical complications that existed before the operation. Patients with preexisting ailments should follow dietary guidelines indicated before surgery unless otherwise indicated by the specialist. Once solids are introduced (~ day 3), liquids and solids should be separated by 30 to 60 minutes. All bariatric procedures typically follow the diet progression and the guidelines listed. Although not all the restrictions are necessary for each procedure, they do assist in healthy eating and weight loss.

Once patients leave the hospital, the recommended progression of food texture varies. Some dietitians recommend liquids for up to 2 weeks; others suggest solids soon after discharge. The typical progression may also vary according to an individual patient's needs. A more conservative approach would be 1 to 2 weeks of liquids, another 1 to 2 weeks of pureed foods, and then a slow advancement to soft textures and regularly textured foods.

Typically, patients can only ingest approximately 1 to 2 oz of intake soon after surgery. Volume will increase with time (this varies from person to person) and should be explained to the patient as being typical. It should also be explained, however, that although volume will increase, it should never resume to "normal." A good indicator that the pouch has stretched is a significant weight gain. A dietary analysis should also be done to verify an

Table 8B.1. Diet Progression During Hospital Stay

Preoperative (24 h Before Surgery)	Day of Surgery (Day 0)	Day 1	Day2	Day 3 (Possible Discharge)	Day 4 (Probable Discharge)
NPO	NPO	Possible introduction of ice chips or water	Clear liquids: Non-carbonated, low-concentrated sugar	Liquids: Non-carbonated, low-concentrated sugar *or* Puree: Noncarbonated, low-concentrated sugar	Liquids: Non-carbonated, low-concentrated sugar *or* Puree: Noncarbonated, low-concentrated sugar *or* Soft: Noncarbonated, low-concentrated sugar
			For example: broth, sugar-free gelatin, diet drinks (sugar substitutes permitted)	For example: broth, sugar-free gelatin, all-natural applesauce, sugar-free yogurt, hot cereal	For example: all-natural applesauce, sugar-free yogurt, hot cereal, scrambled eggs, macaroni, potatoes

increase in food intake. Many clinicians recommend small, frequent feedings soon after surgery, because intake is extremely minimal at this time. If small, frequent feedings cannot be provided in the hospital, it is often recommended that patients keep some nonperishable items at their bedside.

Before discharge, the patient must understand the medical and nutrition guidelines to be followed at home. Written information with a verbal explanation is helpful, as is a contact person for future questions. Patients often do not have questions until solid food is initiated and sometimes feel hopeless if they cannot contact someone. The contact or point person should also be able to triage questions to the appropriate specialist if it is out of his or her scope of practice.

It is also helpful for patients to have contact numbers of other bariatric surgery patients for reference. Many hospitals have contact lists, support groups, on-line support groups, or referrals to support systems. It may also be valuable for some patients to have lists of books and monitored Web sites, for further reference.

Diet Guidelines

Although many patients think of a "diet" in the conventional way of "restriction," it is important to communicate that diet guidelines focus on what patients can eat rather than on what they cannot eat. Of course, foods that are not optimal after surgery (high-calorie, refined sugar–concentrated foods) should be discussed. However, the focus should be on maintaining adequate nutritional status. The point of weight loss for the bariatric patient is to extend life, to minimize or prevent obesity-related complications, and to improve the quality of living.

The approach to weight loss for these individuals is different from all other weight-loss attempts, simply because it is much more difficult to stray from the diet guidelines after one has had surgery. This does not mean, however, that patients always lose weight and/or maintain their weight loss. There are ways to sabotage weight loss even after bariatric surgery (calorie-dense fluids or soft foods like ice cream). The surgery should be thought of as a permanent decision. With this in mind, the active weight-loss phase is only a short period in the person's actual life (6 to 12 months), but the maintenance phase is enduring. Although the weight-loss phase will be the most challenging time for some, the maintenance phase will be the more difficult period for others. It is for this reason that some patients require ongoing nutrition treatment, whereas others require less frequent visits. Often individuals seek nutrition guidance if it is not available through their surgeon's program or hospital.

Because the guidelines are so different from any other type of weight-loss plan, it is essential that the individual understand the nutrition plan that he or she needs to follow. Providing the individual with nutrition education before surgery is recommended, as mentioned in the preoperative section above, and is typically done in most bariatric centers. In the most optimal setting, the guidelines are discussed and provided in written form, so that the patient can review them and refer to them as needed. Some programs provide the nutrition education component in a group setting, which can be helpful to certain types of individuals.

Macronutrients

Protein is encouraged as the primary macronutrient in the bariatric surgery diet, although carbohydrates and fats should not be eliminated. All these nutrients are essential for complete nutrition and should be discussed in terms of foods—not just nutrients. Tables 8B.2, 8B.3, and 8B.4 describe the best-tolerated foods from each of these groups. The lists are most useful during the first few months after surgery, when food intake is new. Most patients discover which foods are best tolerated for them by trial and error. The response

Table 8B.2.   Guidelines for Postoperative Protein Intake

Foods	Easy To Tolerate	Difficult To Tolerate
Meats	Flaky fish, moist chicken (without skin), lean lunch meats, eggs, chopped meat	Shellfish, turkey (if dry), red meat (especially steaks), pork
Dairy	Low fat: yogurt, cottage cheese, soft cheeses, non-fat or low-fat milk	High fat: hard cheeses, ice cream, regular milk, milk shakes, puddings
Legumes, beans, nuts, seeds	All cooked legumes and beans (skins soft or removed), smooth peanut butter or other nut butter, tofu (and other soy products)	All hard nuts, seeds, uncooked legumes or beans, chunky peanut butter
Protein supplements	Low-sugar, low-fat oral supplements in liquid or pudding consistency; powdered protein, powdered milk	High-sugar, high-fat oral supplements; nutrient-enriched bars coated with chocolate or other high-sugar ingredient; bars with a dry consistency or with nuts

Table 8B.3.   Guidelines for Postoperative Carbohydrate Intake

Foods	Easy To Tolerate	Difficult To Tolerate
Vegetables	Cooked vegetables (excluding asparagus, tough skins)	Raw vegetables
Fruits	Bananas, canned fruit in natural juices. (Some people tolerate summer fruits better than winter fruits.)	Dried fruits, hard fruits, skins of fruit, citrus fruits
Breads, pasta	Well-cooked pasta	All types of breads (grainy breads seem to be better tolerated)
Concentrated sugars	None	All concentrated sugars
Crackers, snack foods, other	Minimal	Most

Table 8B.4. Guidelines for Postoperative Fat Intake

Foods	Easy To Tolerate	Difficult To Tolerate
Spreads	Small portions of margarine, low-fat cream cheese, or low-fat mayonnaise	Butter, mayonnaise, cream
Oils	Small amounts of olive, vegetable, and other oils	

to certain foods is quite individual. Some patients have only transient problems tolerating foods; others have some permanent difficulties; still others find no difficulty tolerating most foods. It is nearly impossible to predict in advance those who will have problems and those who will not. It is important to communicate to patients that problems with certain foods may occur.

It is beneficial to provide patients with a list of foods and even a "shopping list" to assist them in making appropriate choices. A high-protein, low-fat supplement is recommended to increase protein intake. Most patients consume 1 to 2 portions (~8 oz) of a supplement daily. This supplement is particularly important during the first 6 months postsurgery, when food intake may not be sufficient.

Side Effects and Monitoring

Dumping syndrome, usually caused by foods such as refined sugars and dense fats, is a concern after gastric bypass surgery. This does not affect patients with restrictive bariatric procedures, such as the vertical banded gastroplasty or the lap band. This syndrome occurs after any operation that alters the normal manner in which food leaves the stomach into the intestines. Basically, the food particles act like sponges, absorbing water into the intestine, which produces a series of symptoms that are usually described as uncomfortable to severely painful. The symptoms of dumping syndrome include lightheadedness, nausea, cold sweats, abdominal cramps, and diarrhea.

Malabsorptive and restrictive procedures, like the gastric bypass, produce the greatest weight loss; however, they can be associated with metabolic and nutritional consequences. Strictly restrictive procedures tend to produce fewer of these complications but have a less desirable weight loss. Nutritional concerns include malnutrition, dehydration, specific vitamin or mineral deficiencies, and weight loss failure.

Nutrition monitoring is especially important during the rapid weight-loss phase, typically the first several months after surgery and longer for some. Weight loss typically stops around 9 to 12 months after surgery. Therefore, careful assessment of the patient's food intake during follow-up visits is important, and diaries are recommended for each meeting. A 3-day food diary appears to be the best method for assessment in this type of setting. Concerns should be communicated to the surgeon and medical physician caring for the patient. If any problems are suspected, immediate contact should be made.

It is typical for patients to have little or no variety in their diets, because of the possibility or fear of a bad reaction. It is important for individuals to try different types of foods, but to do it slowly. It is not uncommon for a patient to have an intolerance one month that resolves the next month. It is also not uncommon for patients to have problems with a food because of the way it was prepared, making the trouble a single incident. If patients are careful and follow the guidelines provided, they tend to have fewer nutrition problems, assuming that there is no metabolic or surgical issue. If a patient has severe intolerances despite following guidelines, he or she should be referred back to the surgeon for further workup.

Nutritional Deficiencies

The most frequently seen, long-term macronutrient problem after gastric surgery is protein deficiency, although this has become less frequent as a result of nutrition education. The complications of inadequate protein should be stressed during the nutrition education sessions and reiterated at follow-up meetings. Deficiency problems include poor wound healing, loss of lean body mass, and possibly hair loss (although this is often attributed to rapid weight loss). Protein should be encouraged and monitored at counseling sessions. Most patients do not ingest the recommended protein intake in the first few months after surgery with diet alone. Protein supplements are suggested for this reason.

The most frequently seen, long-term micronutrient problems after gastric surgery are iron, vitamin B-12, folate, and calcium deficiencies (1). In one series, the frequency of vitamin B-12 deficiency was 70%; folate, <5%; and iron, 70% (2). These deficiencies are attributed to reduced gastric acidity in the partitioned stomach, in combination with reduced absorption due to bypassing the small intestine and not due to change in intrinsic factor secretion (3). Compliance with recommended vitamin/mineral supplements is essential during weight loss and weight maintenance. Oral intake will always be minimal, and the intestine and stomach will remain bypassed despite weight maintenance. If noncompliance is suspected, communication with the physician is recommended.

Supplements

Typically, an adult multivitamin or two children's multivitamins (chewable) are recommended. Some patients choose to take a liquid vitamin instead. In addition, vitamin B-12 is required either by a monthly shot or daily sublingual tablets (a nasal spray is also available). Patients who do not have a malabsorptive procedure do not need additional B-12. Additional iron is also recommended, 325 mg ferrous sulfate, most especially for menstruating women. Also recommended are 1 mg of folate and 1,000 to 1,500 mg of calcium citrate, to prevent osteoporosis, because malabsorption of calcium has been noted. If a micronutrient deficiency is indicated, either through blood work or nutrition assessment, additional supplementation is recommended to minimize the specific deficiency.

It is recommended that the patient visit the registered dietitian often (several times after surgery and then typically monthly as needed), to ensure adequate nutritional status. The registered dietitian should communicate with the surgeon and medical physician, who may not see the patient as often. Patients who are unable to visit the dietitian regularly should attend support groups run by professionals.

Food intakes change markedly, in part because of diet counseling, but also because of anatomic changes from the gastric partitioning procedure and the potential for dumping syndrome to occur. In one series, preoperative caloric intake was reported at 2,600 to 3,100 kcal/day, and dropped to 1,400 to 1,750 kcal/day 4 years after surgery (2). A second series found significantly lower caloric intake and reduced enjoyment of calorically dense foods after the gastric bypass procedure (4). It is not uncommon for patients to report aversions to once-preferred foods, including problems with aromas and visual cues. It is essential that patients do not limit themselves drastically, diminishing variety in their diet, and increasing their risk for nutritional deficiencies.

Dehydration

Dehydration may also be seen after surgery and must be addressed. Dehydration occurs more frequently in the first few months after surgery and in the warmer months. The patient's requirement to maintain normal fluid balance is not changed after surgery and therefore can be a challenge with the restricted gastric capacity. Calorie-free liquids, with an emphasis on water, should be encouraged throughout the day. Liquids can include ice chips and low-calorie, low-sugar ice pops. If vomiting and diarrhea also occur, fluid derangement may be severely exacerbated. Once dehydrated, patients have a difficult time rehydrating adequately, because they cannot take in fluids quickly. Intravenous fluids may be required for some patients, to restore lost intravascular volume.

Inadequate Weight Loss

Weight-loss failures also occur after gastric surgery. Minimal weight loss or even weight gain can occur. This may be due to dietary noncompliance, although gastric capacity has also been related to weight-loss failure (5). Patients who chronically abuse calorically dense foods and/or overeat will usually not lose a significant amount of weight. With time, this behavior can cause pouch dilation or staple line disruption (6). This usually would require reoperation to initiate weight loss once again.

Case Study. John

John enters your office with a 50-lb weight gain in 6 weeks. After surgery 2 years ago, he lost 130 lb. He is extremely concerned, because he finds himself hungry all the time and is able to eat large portions without feeling satisfied or uncomfortable. He is trying to watch his diet but is finding that he can eat all types of foods. He needs your help. After reviewing John's diet carefully, you find that he is eating unusually large amounts of food for a gastric bypass patient. He has probably stretched his pouch, thus causing the weight gain, lack of fullness, and ability to eat large portions. At this point, healthy food choices should be recommended, to minimize any further weight gain. Discuss whether John would like to contact his surgeon. Even if John would not consider reoperation, he should contact his surgeon to determine whether he needs to be seen. If John would reconsider reoperation, preoperative nutrition guidelines should be discussed once again, close to the surgery date.

Weight Loss and Exercise

Weight loss after the gastric bypass procedure is typically greater than with the vertical banded gastroplasty and other restrictive procedures. There has been significant documentation of weight loss results after a variety of procedures (See Part A of this chapter). In one study of more than 5,300 patients, an overall weight loss of 50% to 64% of excess body weight was reported after 6 years (7). In another study, a weight loss of 62% of excess weight of the sample studied was maintained after 4 years (8); and in yet another study, a weight loss of more than 50% of excess weight was maintained after 14 years (5). It is obvious from these results and many other studies that surgery can induce significant weight loss (see Part A of this chapter). Exact weight loss is difficult to predict; however, it can be enhanced not only with a healthful diet but also with exercise.

Exercise is a key element to successful weight loss and maintenance for the bariatric patient. Often individuals believe that exercise is unnecessary, because the surgery will cause weight loss regardless of activity. The benefits of exercise should be incorporated into the nutrition education and should not be underestimated by the clinician or the patient (see Chapter 6: Physical Activity). Patients may experience fatigue for several weeks after surgery, but gradually stamina improves and energy returns to normal. Minimal activity begins in the hospital, to prevent pneumonia, blood clots, and constipation, as indicated earlier. A continual progression of activity will only enhance weight-loss efforts by burning calories. As weight loss increases, activity will become easier for the individual who may have trouble in the beginning. It is important, however, that the patient does not initiate an exercise plan until the surgeon and medical physicians believe activity is appropriate and safe for the individual.

Final Note

Although much work remains in the field of nutrition guidelines for the bariatric surgery patient, there is much we do know based on observation and experiences from former procedures. Surgeons are refining their techniques in bariatric surgery, and nutrition professionals are continually improving the guidelines for these high-risk patients. It is an area that has made considerable strides in an extremely short period of time. Although there are still many clinical and research questions to be resolved, it is apparent that optimal health after surgery is possible when there is a focus on nutrition as a major part of treatment.

References

1. Brolin RE, Gorman JH, Gorman RC, Petschenik AJ, Bradley LJ, Kenler HA, Cody RP. Are vitamin B12 and folate deficiency clinically important after roux-en-Y gastric bypass? *J Gastrointest Surg*.1998;2:436–442.
2. Brolin RL, Robertson LB, Kenler HA, Cody RP. Weight loss and dietary intake after vertical banded gastroplasty and Roux-en-Y gastric bypass. *Ann Surg*. 1994;220:782–790.
3. Rhode BM, Arseneau P, Cooper BA, Katz M, Gilfix BM, MacLean LD. Vitamin B-12 deficiency after gastric surgery for obesity. *Am J Clin Nutr*. 1996; 63:103–109.
4. Halmi KA, Mason E, Falk JR, Stunkard A. Appetitive behavior after gastric bypass for obesity. *Int J Obes*. 1981;5:457–464.
5. Pories WJ, Swanson MS, MacDonald KG, Long SB, Morris PG, Brown BM, Barakat HA, deRamon RA, Israel G, Dolzal JM. Who would have thought it?

An operation proves to be the most effective therapy for adult-onset diabetes mellitus. *Ann Surg.* 1995;222:339–350.

6. Shikora SA. Surgical treatment for severe obesity: the state of the art for the new millennium. *Nutr Clin Pract.* 2000;15:13–22.

7. Benotti PN, Hollingshead J, Mascioli EA, Bothe A Jr, Bistrian BR, Blackburn GL. Gastric restrictive operations for morbid obesity. *Am J Surg.*1989;157: 150–155.

8. Capella JF, Capella RF. The weight reduction operation choice: vertical banded gastroplasty or gastric bypass? *Am J Surg.* 1996;171:74–79.

Chapter 9
Weight-Loss Maintenance

PART A. Overview

Rena R. Wing, PhD

Maintenance of weight loss remains a major problem in the treatment of obesity. On average, participants in behavioral weight-loss programs will lose 9 kg (8% to 10% of their weight) during the first 6 months of treatment and will maintain approximately two thirds of this initial weight loss (5 to 6 kg) at 1-year follow-up (1). Despite intensive efforts, weight regain appears to continue for the next several years (2). Maintenance of a 4% weight loss at year 4 follow-up has been reported (3), but other studies suggest that by 5 years participants are back to baseline weight (4).

This section will address two approaches to increasing the understanding of long-term maintenance of weight loss. The first approach is to study those clients successful in weight-loss maintenance, to learn how they accomplished this feat. The second is to study the outcomes of randomized clinical trials that used specific strategies aimed at improving maintenance of weight loss (5).

The National Weight Control Registry

The National Weight Control Registry (NWCR), an ongoing study of individuals who have been successful at long-term maintenance of weight loss, was started in 1994 by Drs. James Hill and Rena Wing (5). To enter the Registry, participants must be older than 18 years, must have lost at least 30 lb, and must have maintained a 30-lb weight loss for more than 1 year. Currently, there are more than 3,000 individuals in the registry. These individuals have lost 60 lb on average (reducing from a body mass index [BMI] of 36.3 to 24.9) and have maintained their weight loss for more than 6 years. Key findings from the Registry are listed below:

- Those successful have tried to lose weight many times before—but unsuccessfully. Thus, there is nothing inherently different between those unsuccessful and those successful in weight loss. Stated differently, individuals who are unsuccessful can become successful in weight loss. The variables that appeared to distinguish the successful effort from earlier attempts were a greater level of commitment, a stricter diet, and a greater reliance on exercise (6).
- Individuals successful at weight loss used a variety of approaches. Approximately half received help from a structured program, a registered dietitian, or a physician, whereas the other half lost weight entirely on their own (6). Although a variety of approaches were used for weight loss, certain characteristics were common to the experience of maintaining the weight loss.
- NWCR members consistently report consuming a low-calorie, low-fat diet (1,400 kcal/day, with 24% of calories from fat). Fewer than 1% report consuming a low-carbohydrate regimen, similar to what would be recommended by the Atkins diet (5).
- NWCR members report regular eating, with 5 eating episodes per day. Most (78%) report consuming breakfast on a daily basis (7). They continue to dine out, but they limit fast-food meals to fewer than 1 per week (.74 times per week), on average (6).
- To maintain weight loss, physical activity and diet are used in combination. On average, NWCR members report approximately 2,800 kcal per week of physical activity. That would be equivalent to walking 28 miles per week (4 miles per day) or 60 to 90 minutes of activity per day (5). Walking was the most popular form of exercise, but cycling, weight lifting, and aerobics were also frequently indicated.
- Maintaining weight loss appears to require ongoing vigilance. Most NWCR members (75%) weigh themselves at least weekly; they also exhibit high levels of dietary restraint, similar to those actually losing weight (8).
- More than 90% of NWCR members report that their weight loss has improved their quality of life, level of energy, mobility, general mood, and self-confidence (6).

Randomized Clinical Trials

The NWCR includes a large number of highly successful individuals. However, it should be noted that the NWCR consists of a self-selected population and may not be representative of all individuals successful in weight loss. Methodologically, randomized clinical trials are a stronger way to define the variables associated with long-term weight loss.

Intensive, Ongoing Contact

Maintenance of weight loss is improved by providing regular treatment contact. Perri et al (9) compared 20-week and 40-week behavioral treatment programs. They found that lengthening the treatment led to greater weight losses and delayed the onset of weight regain. Similarly, after a 6-month treatment program, patients who continued to see professionals biweekly throughout the following year had improved long-term outcomes (10).

Exercise

Many studies compare diet alone, exercise alone, and the combination of diet and exercise (11). These studies are quite consistent in showing that the best long-term weight losses use a combination of diet and exercise (12). In fact, the clearest benefit of exercise appears to be for the maintenance of weight loss. Exercising at home (rather than in supervised settings) (13) and providing treadmills for home use (14) both appear to improve maintenance of exercise and consequently weight loss. To date, no differences in maintenance of weight loss have been reported from aerobic exercise, strength training, or the combination of these two approaches (15,16).

Recently, attention has focused on the ideal amount of exercise for maintenance of weight loss (see Chapter 6: Physical Activity). Typically, behavioral treatment programs recommend 1,000 kcal per week of activity. However, on the basis of the NWCR and several other studies, investigators have suggested that higher levels of exercise might be preferable. Jeffery and Wing (17) compared weight loss in participants randomly assigned to 1,000 or 2,500 kcal per week of exercise. The higher exercise dose was associated with greater weight losses at 12 and 18 months, but even at the higher dose of exercise, maximum weight losses were achieved at 12 months, followed by weight regain.

Diet

Most studies of dietary interventions have focused on initial weight loss rather than maintenance. Very-low-calorie diets (diets of 400 kcal per day of lean meat, fish, and fowl, or liquid formula) were found to markedly improve initial weight losses (20 kg weight loss after 12 weeks), but the magnitude of weight regain was greater than on more-balanced, low-calorie regimens (18). Consequently, at the end of 12 to 24 months, there was typically no difference between the two approaches.

Enhancing the structure of the diet may improve long-term results. Participants who were given the actual food they should eat or were given structured meal plans and grocery lists achieved larger weight losses than those on the same calorie level but following a self-selected diet (19,20). Of particular note for the maintenance of weight loss is a 4-year trial involving SlimFast (21). Patients who were randomly assigned to use 2 SlimFast per day and a healthy dinner lost more weight than patients on a self-selected diet at the same calorie level; moreover, the SlimFast group retained their weight losses better during 4 years of follow-up.

Problem Solving

Although ongoing treatment contact is important, it has remained unclear exactly what should occur at these sessions. Recently, Perri et al (22) compared a group given no maintenance contact with two groups given maintenance programs—one that focused on relapse prevention and one that focused on problem solving. Both the relapse and problem-solving groups met biweekly for a year. The problem-solving group produced the best long-term weight loss, maintaining a weight loss of 10.8 kg at 17 months. The relapse-prevention group maintained a weight loss that averaged 5.8 kg, and the behavioral program (with no maintenance contact) maintained a weight loss of 4.1 kg.

Social Support

To improve maintenance of weight loss, it may be important to increase social support for diet and exercise changes. Involving friends and family members who will be available after the treatment program has ended should be particularly effective. Wing and Jeffery studied two types of social support (23). The first, natural support, was examined by comparing participants who joined a weight-loss program alone vs those who joined the program along with 3 friends. Social support was induced through the use of intragroup cohesiveness activities and intergroup competitions. Both the natural and experimentally created support affected the outcome. The highest number of individuals who completed the study, as well as those with the best maintenance of weight loss, occurred in those patients who entered the program with their friends and were treated in a program with a high level of experimentally created social support.

Increasing Initial Weight Loss vs Setting Modest Weight-Loss Goals

Several studies have explored the potential benefits of setting modest weight-loss goals for participants. Participants often expect to lose more weight during treatment than is reasonable (24) and thus may be disappointed by their outcome (and hence likely to regain). Researchers have therefore tried to help patients to accept more "reasonable" weight-loss goals. Such programs have not been fully evaluated, but preliminary data suggest that setting lower expectations appears to decrease weight loss (25). In contrast, in post hoc analyses, Jeffery, Wing, and Mayer (26) have shown that the more patients lose initially, the better their long-term results. Thus, aggressive approaches that maximize initial weight loss appear to be more effective for long-term weight loss, although removing patients from all foods with very-low-calorie diet regimens is not effective in the long term.

The Future of Weight-Loss Maintenance

Helping patients to maintain their weight loss long-term is one of the most important issues in the field of obesity. To address this issue, it is important to first determine what makes maintenance of weight loss so difficult. Participants appear to be able to lose weight successfully for about 6 months but then begin to regain. The timing of weight regain appears to be similar in most cases, despite differences in the magnitude of weight loss, which suggests that psychological or motivational factors may be operant, rather than physiological changes. Randomized controlled trials are needed (1) to examine strategies for enhancing participant motivation long-term, (2) to determine whether it is necessary to modify preferences for healthy foods and physical activity in order to sustain weight loss, and (3) to investigate novel approaches to encouraging adherence to the behavior changes required for long-term maintenance of weight loss.

Conclusion

The NWCR provides evidence that it is possible to lose significant amounts of weight and maintain the weight loss long-term. The key strategies for weight-loss maintenance appear to be consumption of a low-calorie, low-fat diet; high levels of physical activity; and remaining vigilant about one's weight.

Similar findings occur in randomized controlled trials on weight-loss maintenance. In such studies, the maximum weight loss typically occurs at

6 to 12 months, followed by weight regain. Maintenance of weight loss has been improved, however, by maximizing contact with participants, including high levels of exercise within the intervention, providing structured approaches to dietary intake, increasing social support and problem-solving techniques, and increasing initial weight-loss success.

References

1. Wing RR. Behavioral approaches to the treatment of obesity. In: Bray GH, Bouchard C, James WPT, eds. *Handbook of Obesity.* New York, NY: Marcel Dekker; 1998:855–873.
2. Knowler WC, Barrett-Conner E, Fowler SE, Hamman RF, Lachin JM, Walker EA, Nathan DM. Reduction in the incidence of type 2 diabetes with lifestyle intervention or metformin. *N Engl J Med.* 2002;346:393–403.
3. Kramer FM, Jeffery RW, Forster JL, Snell MK. Long-term follow-up of behavioral treatment for obesity: patterns of weight regain among men and women. *Int J Obes.* 1989;13:123–136.
4. Wadden TA, Sternberg JA, Letizia KA, Stunkard AJ, Foster GD. Treatment of obesity by very low calorie diet, behavior therapy, and their combination: a five-year perspective. *Int J Obes.*1989;13:39–46.
5. Wing RR, Hill JO. Successful weight loss maintenance. *Ann Rev Nutr.* 2001; 21:323–341.
6. Klem ML, Wing RR, McGuire MT, Seagle HM, Hill JO. A descriptive study of individuals successful at long-term maintenance of substantial weight loss. *Am J Clin Nutr.* 1997;66:239–246.
7. Wyatt HR, Grunwald GK, Mosca CL, Klem ML, Wing RR, Hill JO. Long-term weight loss and breakfast in subjects in the National Weight Control Registry. *Obes Res.* 2002;10:78–82.
8. Klem ML, Wing RR, McGuire MT, Seagle HM, Hill JO. Psychological symptoms in individuals successful at long-term maintenance of weight loss. *Health Psychol.* 1998;17:336–345.
9. Perri MG, Nezu AM, Patti ET, McCann KL. Effect of length of treatment on weight loss. *J Consult Clin Psychol.* 1989;57:450–452.
10. Perri MG, McAllister DA, Gange JJ, Jordan RC, McAdoo WG, Nezu AM. Effects of four maintenance programs on the long-term management of obesity. *J Clin Psychol.* 1988;56:529–534.
11. National Institutes of Health. Clinical guidelines on the identification, evaluation, and treatment of overweight and obesity in adults-The evidence report. *Obes Res.* 1998;6(Suppl 2):51S–210S.
12. Wing RR. Physical activity in the treatment of the adulthood overweight and obesity: current evidence and research issues. *Med Sci Sports Exerc.* 1999; 31(11 Suppl):S547–S552.
13. Perri MG, Martin AD, Leermakers EA, Sears SF, Notelavitz M. Effects of group- versus home-based exercise in the treatment of obesity. *J Consult Clin Psychol.* 1997;65:278–285.

14. Jakicic JM, Winters C, Lang W, Wing RR. Effects of intermittent exercise and use of home exercise equipment on adherence, weight loss, and fitness in overweight women. *JAMA.* 1999;282:1554–1560.

15. Wadden TA, Vogt RA, Andersen RE, Bartlett SJ, Foster GD, Kuehnel RH, Wilk J, Weinstock R, Buckenmeyer P, Berkowitz RI, Steen SN. Exercise in the treatment of obesity: effects of four interventions on body composition, resting energy expenditure, appetite, and mood. *J Consult Clin Psychol.* 1997;65: 269–277.

16. Wadden TA, Vogt RA, Foster GD, Anderson DA. Exercise and maintenance of weight loss: 1-year follow-up of a controlled clinic trial. *J Consult Clin Psychol.* 1998;66:429–433.

17. Jeffery RW, Wing RW. The effects of an enhanced exercise program on long-term weight loss [abstract]. *Obes Res.* 2001;9(Suppl 3):100S.

18. National Task Force on the Prevention and Treatment of Obesity. Very low calorie diets. *JAMA.* 1993;270:967–974.

19. Jeffery RW, Wing RR, Thorson C, Burton LR, Raether C, Harvey J, Mullen M. Strengthening behavioral interventions for weight loss: a randomized trial of food provision and monetary incentives. *J Consult Clin Psychol.* 1993;61: 1038–1045.

20. Wing RR, Jeffery RW, Burton LR, Thorson C, Nissinoff KS, Baxter JE. Food provision vs structured meal plans in the behavioral treatment of obesity. *Int J Obes Metab Disord.* 1996;20:56–62.

21. Flechtner-Mors M, Ditschuneit HH, Johnson TD, Suchard MA, Adler G. Metabolic and weight loss effects of long-term dietary intervention in obese patients: four-year results. *Obes Res.* 2000;8:399–402.

22. Perri MG, Nezu AM, McKelvey WF, Shermer RL, Renjilian DA, Viegener BJ. Relapse prevention training and problem-solving therapy in the long-term management of obesity. *J Consult Clin Psychol.* 2001;69:722–726.

23. Wing RR, Jeffery RW. Benefits of recruiting participants with friends and increasing social support for weight loss maintenance. *J Consult Clin Psychol.* 1999;67:132–138.

24. Foster GD, Wadden TA, Vogt RA, Brewer G. What is a reasonable weight loss? Patients' expectations and evaluations of obesity treatment outcomes. *J Consult Clin Psychol.* 1997;65:79–85.

25. Phelan S, Foster G, Wadden TA, Gill D, Ermold J, Didie E. Improving body image and self-esteem in obese women. Abstract presented at: Annual meeting of the Society of Behavioral Medicine; March 2001; Seattle, Wash.

26. Jeffery RW, Wing RR, Mayer RR. Are smaller weight losses or more achievable weight loss goals better in the long term for obese patients? *J Consult Clin Psychol.* 1998;66:641–645.

PART B. Practical Applications

Suzanne Phelan, PhD

Practical Guidelines for Weight Maintenance

Weight loss and weight maintenance share many requisite behaviors, including consuming a reduced-calorie diet, increasing physical activity, and practicing behavioral strategies. A critical difference between the two processes, however, is the presence of motivators. During weight loss, patients experience a variety of motivating factors: weekly feedback from the scale; compliments from others about their weight loss; and noticeable improvements in mood, energy, body image, and health. During weight maintenance, however, many of these advantages disappear: compliments decline, the scale doesn't budge, adherence becomes more challenging, and the improvements in health become less salient. In such a context, it is difficult for patients to maintain their weight loss. This section describes specific strategies to help patients achieve successful weight-loss maintenance, including methods to reverse weight regain and to increase patient motivation during challenging times.

Skills That Promote Weight Maintenance

Patients who have lost weight already know the skills required for weight control. The goal now is to facilitate their continued practice of weight-control behaviors and to help them take ownership of these behaviors for life.

For example, a patient has lost 10% of her initial body weight by eating a low-calorie diet, exercising, and consistent self-monitoring of eating and activity. Although, ideally, she would like to lose more weight, she is now willing to work at weight maintenance because she "can't imagine" consuming less or exercising more than she already does. It is clear that the patient is well educated about energy balance, exercise, self-monitoring, and other behavioral strategies. Now what? What can be done to keep her engaged in the treatment process and to help her remain successful at weight maintenance?

Frequent Patient-Provider Contact

As stated in the Overview section of this chapter, frequent contact between the patient and the provider appears critical during the maintenance period (1).

Contact every 2 weeks is recommended. However, at a minimum, monthly visits should be maintained, and more frequent contact should be scheduled when patients begin to regain weight.

Ironically, when patients are at greatest risk for weight regain (ie, when the maintenance stage begins), contact with treatment providers tends to decline. Some treatment programs finish when maintenance starts. More often, however, patients gradually drop out of the treatment process by missing treatment visits or by not returning phone calls. Patients may stop attending treatment for a variety of reasons, including financial limitations, feeling bored with the treatment process, or feeling ready to "do it on their own" now that they have lost weight. However, it is generally safe to assume that patients who start reducing contact are doing poorly.

There are several different ways to maintain contact with patients after weight loss. Although bimonthly visits with a practitioner is the ideal, this option may not be affordable for some patients. Another strategy is for patients to attend community weight-loss groups on a bimonthly basis, with individual meetings with the practitioner on a quarterly basis. This method can offset treatment costs for the patient while providing both group and individual support. Alternatively, telephone check-ins or e-mail contacts with the practitioner can be used in conjunction with quarterly face-to-face visits. This provides a fast and practical means of maintaining contact with the patient; however, some patients may not have easy access to a computer. Other members of the practitioner's staff can also help maintain contact with the patient. Staff may provide bimonthly "check-ins" or may be available for weigh-ins at the clinic, while individual visits with the patient's primary provider are scheduled on a quarterly basis.

Regular Weighing

In addition to being weighed at each treatment visit, the practitioner should encourage patients to weigh themselves at home on a daily basis. The rationale for frequent weighing is that it keeps patients attentive to their weight and gives them the information they need to make quick adjustments. When patients step on the scale daily, they are able to make shifts in their eating and exercise immediately when their weight begins to creep up past their maintenance level. Daily weighing also allows patients to identify weight changes due to transient shifts in salt and water intake vs changes in fat stores.

Regular Physical Activity

A patient's level of physical activity should also be monitored at each clinical encounter. Patients working at weight maintenance are likely already engaged in some form of physical activity. The goal during maintenance is to increase the duration of exercise. At a minimum, patients should be encouraged to accumulate 30 minutes of moderate-intensity physical activity (equivalent to brisk walking) 5 days per week. Once they are comfortable with this minimum level, they should continue to strive to increase their goal to 300 to 400 minutes per week (1 hour per day, 5 to 7 days per week). There are a variety of strategies that can be used to promote higher levels of activity during maintenance. (Several of the following items are discussed in greater detail in Chapter 6: Physical Activity.)

Self-Monitoring.   Most patients who have lost weight in standard treatment programs are familiar with self-monitoring—"too familiar," some will say. Until the physical activity goal is reached, it is helpful for patients to continue recording their minutes of activity each day, counting anything that is equivalent to brisk walking and that lasts 10 minutes or more. Once patients have reached their exercise goal, self-monitoring may be reduced to 1 to 2 weeks per month, providing a way for patients to ensure that a high level of physical activity is maintained.

Pedometer.   Purchasing a pedometer and recording the number of steps taken each day, with 10,000 steps per day being the ultimate goal, is also helpful for promoting tracking increases in lifestyle activity.

Enjoyable Activities.   Encourage patients to choose activities that they enjoy. If they enjoy an activity, they may be more likely to continue doing it.

Variety.   Some patients find that by keeping the same exercise routine, it is easier for them to stay on track. This style works because once they determine their routine, they do not have to think about it as much; it becomes a part of their daily life. For other people, however, variety keeps them motivated. They find it boring to follow the same routine over and over again, and doing a variety of different exercises actually helps them stay on track. Patients who report feeling bored with their exercise may benefit from adding a new variation of activity (eg, instead of taking their usual aerobics class, they can try spinning) or trying a new activity altogether (eg, taking a lesson in something they have always dreamed about, such as ice skating or rock climbing). Of the successful members of the National Weight Control Registry (NWCR), many reported walking as their primary activity; however, many combined walking with other activities (2). Table 9B.1 lists the six most-frequent activities reported by NWCR participants.

Reduced-Calorie, Low-Fat Diet

As noted earlier, the successful members of NWCR clearly ate a low-calorie diet (women 843 to 1,750 kcal/day, and men 1,078 to 2,372 kcal/day) that

Table 9B.1. Activities Reported by Successful
Weight Losers of the National Weight Control Registry

Activity	Those Reporting To Participate in the Activity (%)
Walking	76.6
Cycling	20.6
Weight lifting	20.3
Aerobics	17.8
Running	10.5
Stair climbing	9.3

Data are from reference 2.

was also low in fat (24% calories from fat). How many calories should patients who are working at weight maintenance eat? The answer to this question depends on the patient's goal. If the patient's goal is truly to maintain weight, the average number of calories eaten each day is a good reference point for what the body needs to stay at its current weight. Given that most patients underreport their dietary intake, however, their reported calorie intake should be considered only an estimate of their actual intake (3). If the patient desires to continue losing weight, it is useful to provide fixed-calorie diets of 1,200 kcal/day for patients weighing less than 200 lb, and 1,500 kcal/day for patients weighing more than 200 lb.

Unfortunately, there are many barriers to maintaining a reduced-calorie, low-fat diet. Patients may report craving fast foods, feeling bored with their diet, feeling deprived, or questioning whether they can eat fewer calories long-term. Under such pressure, attention to calories and portion sizes may wane. There are several strategies, however, to help patients remain attentive to their dietary intake and to continue to consume a low-fat, reduced-calorie diet.

Self-Monitoring. Similar to the self-monitoring of exercise; patients should keep records of their calorie intake until they have reached their weight-maintenance goal. After their goal is reached, individuals should engage in periodic self-monitoring (eg, in response to small weight gains), to ensure that small changes in the diet do not go unnoticed. Consider simplifying the self-monitoring process during maintenance. For example, a patient who consumes one of three different breakfasts on a regular basis could identify, in advance, the portion size and calorie content of breakfast 1, breakfast 2, and breakfast 3. To record, the patient would simply write the number corresponding to the breakfast selection, rather than list the portions and calorie content of the breakfast's individual items. Creating checklists that itemize different food selections may also help simplify recording during maintenance.

Dietary Variety. Some patients find that by eating the same foods over and over, it is easier for them to stay on track with their eating. Other patients find that eating the same thing day after day becomes boring. Patients who have reached a weight-loss plateau after 6 months of dieting, for example, may report feeling bored with their current dietary regimen. In such cases, adding a little variety to the diet may offset feelings of boredom. The practitioner may explore with such patients which meals or snacks are causing boredom and suggest ways to alter the particular eating situation (eg, change breakfast cereals). Practitioners may also encourage patients to explore new vegetables and fruit (eg, turnips, okra, parsnips, rutabaga, star fruit, or cactus pears) or to try new low-calorie recipes.

Dietary Novelty. Sometimes, a more dramatic change in the dietary regimen is needed to keep patients captivated and therefore mindful of dietary intake. For example, if a patient is consuming a standard, self-selected diet, the practitioner can provide guidelines for a vegetarian diet for 6 months, followed by a Mediterranean-type diet. Alternatively, meal replacements and prepackaged frozen entrees may be incorporated into the diet. For example, a patient may consume self-selected foods for breakfast, snacks, and dinner but consume a meal replacement for lunch. Meal replacements are highly recommended for patients who start to regain weight (as described below).

Problem Solving

Problem solving is another useful tool for weight maintenance (4). Practitioners promoting weight maintenance should remind patients of the basic steps of problem solving and revisit this skill on an ongoing basis throughout treatment. Problem solving is helpful in identifying solutions to current, past, or future problems related to eating and exercise. Problem solving can be broken down into three steps.

1. *Defining the Problem.* The more specific the patient can be in identifying the problem, the easier it will be to identify solutions. Patients should think carefully about when a particular problem started. Many times an exercise lapse or an episode of overeating is at the end of a long chain of problematic behaviors (see Chapter 4: Behavioral Treatment). For example, if a patient reports eating a box of cookies, the practitioner should query about how the box of cookies got into the house in the first place.

To define the problem, practitioners should help patients identify the source, or beginning, of the problematic behavior chain.

2. *Brainstorming Possible Solutions.* Once patients have identified the problem, the next step is to think about all possible solutions to the problem. Perhaps exercise has declined because it is getting dark earlier and the patient does not want to walk alone at night. Some possible solutions could include exercising in the morning, finding a walking partner, exercising at a shopping mall, or taking a walk during the lunch hour. Many more options could be generated. At this stage, patients should be encouraged to think about all possible solutions, not just the ones that seem most realistic or feasible.

3. *Implementing One of the Solutions.* From the list of possible solutions, pick a solution that the patient thinks would work best and then try it. Future sessions should then revisit the issue and evaluate whether the solution has worked. If it has not, another strategy from the list should be implemented. This process should be repeated until the patient is successful.

Anticipating High-Risk Situations

Another important skill for patients working at weight maintenance is to identify and anticipate high-risk situations. These include situational or emotional triggers that increase a patient's risk of overeating and/or inactivity.

Situational Triggers.   Vacations and holidays are, perhaps, the most obvious examples of situational triggers for relapse. Some patients choose to lose a few pounds to create a "buffer" before the impending high-risk period. A goal, for example, could be to lose 4 lb during the month preceding a vacation or holiday. In order to do this, patients would need a 3,500-kcal deficit, or an energy deficit of 500 kcal per day to lose 1 lb per week. Other triggers for overeating may include places (eg, restaurants) or people (eg, relatives). After such high-risk situations are identified, problem solving may be used to prevent them from developing into weight regain.

Emotional Triggers.   It is particularly important for practitioners working with patients maintaining their weight to monitor levels of stress and negative affect. Greater depressive symptoms and stress commonly precede weight regain (5,6). Thus, helping patients develop strategies to reduce the potential adverse effects of mood and stress on eating and exercise is critical. Ideally, patients are able to anticipate when stress or dysphoria will occur (eg, during holidays or a particular time of year at work). Problem solving may be used to identify the specific factors that are likely to trigger regain and the strategies to cope effectively with the upcoming situation.

However, more often the patient experiencing an increase in stress or negative mood will start missing treatment sessions. In these cases, it is important for the practitioner to try to maintain contact with the patient (eg, by e-mail or telephone) and use these opportunities to provide support and help with problem solving. Patients reporting clinically significant distress should be referred to a mental health professional.

Coping With Lapse and Relapse

Inevitably, patients will have times when they eat amounts of food that they do not consider appropriate for long-term weight loss. Bob arrives at the treatment session with a look of guilt on his face. The scale is up a few pounds, and he feels terrible about it. While Bob continues to weigh himself frequently and to exercise, his eating has been out of control after an incident at work left him feeling angry.

Before such occasions become more frequent, strategies to prevent the lapse from turning into a relapse need to be implemented. In this section, strategies for coping with lapse (ie, a temporary setback) and relapse (ie, a significant weight regain) are reviewed. These strategies, as well as strategies to prevent weight regain, are summarized in Table 9B.2.

Table 9B.2. Strategies for Weight Maintenance, Coping with Lapse, and Coping with Relapse

Weight Status	Strategies
Maintenance	Frequent patient-provider contact Frequent weighing High level of physical activity Low-calorie, low-fat diet Problem solving Anticipating high-risk situations
Lapse (3–4 lb higher than starting maintenance weight)	Problem solving Stop negative thinking Develop a plan
Relapse (≥ 5 lb above starting maintenance weight)	Simplify the dietary regimen Meal replacements Structured meal plans Self-monitoring Consider medication

Responding to a Lapse

Patients who are experiencing a lapse typically have not reverted completely back to their former eating and exercise habits. They have experienced a minor setback that can be remedied with some immediate intervention. Here are a few strategies that can help patients get back on track.

Putting the Lapse in Perspective. First, practitioners should help patients to recognize that they are not alone; everyone experiences lapses. The key is to recognize that a lapse has occurred and to take steps quickly to remedy the situation.

Promoting Realistic Thinking. The second step in recovering from a lapse is to help the patient resist the tendency toward negative thoughts and feelings. After a lapse, some patients may say to themselves "I'm a failure," "I'll never succeed," or "I blew it; why even try." Such distorted thinking can lead to feelings of discouragement, guilt, and/or anger at being in this position "once again." It is important to identify such thoughts and feelings, because they can undermine a patient's ability to deal effectively with a lapse. Such thinking should be countered by more realistic thoughts about the situation and the patient's success. The person who "blew it" today is the same person who has been successful during many previous weeks. A lapse in behavior is not revealing "the real them." It is simply another occasion of eating behavior from which they can recover and learn.

The first step to learning from the situation is to look closely at it and to ask what led to inappropriate eating. Often, lapses coincide with a specific high-risk situation (eg, argument at work, holidays). In such cases, efforts can be made to alter the high-risk situation (eg, bringing low-calorie foods to a holiday party) or the patient's reactions to it (eg, assertiveness training for interpersonal distress, relaxation techniques). If the situation was temporary, such as a holiday or a wedding, once the patient is back in the usual environment, eating and exercise habits may normalize.

Sometimes lapses are the result of a series of subtle behavior changes that are going unnoticed (Table 9B.3). Alone, each of these small behaviors may not result in any weight change; accumulated, they may account for a lapse. The key is to recognize the snowball effect. With time these small behaviors can accumulate and lead to a loss of control of weight maintenance.

Regaining Control. The third step is to regain control of eating or exercise at the very next opportunity. Encourage patients to avoid self-statements such as, "Well, I blew it for the day," and waiting until the next day to start controlling their behavior. It is best to make the very next meal a controlled one or to make the next opportunity a time to be active. This strategy helps keep lapses in perspective—as temporary setbacks.

Table 9B.3. Behavioral Changes That Contribute to a Lapse

Behavior During Successful Weight Control	Sign of Lapse
Adding nonfat milk to coffee	Adding cream to coffee
Putting jelly on toast	Putting butter on toast
Ordering dressing on the side	Not specifying orders at restaurants
Parking farther away at shopping malls	Parking as close as possible to the door
Exercising 30 min, 5 d/wk	Exercising 15 min, 5 d/wk

Responding to a Relapse

Despite all best efforts, some patients may end up eating inappropriately on a string of occasions or not exercising for a long period of time, and significant weight regain is the result. At this point, immediate action is necessary to get back on track. Reducing calorie intake should be the focus, because it is hard to suddenly increase exercise enough to make a real difference in energy balance. One of the most effective ways to reverse weight regain is to simplify choices and to provide structure. There are several options that may be considered, alone or in combination, to reduce calorie intake.

Self-Monitoring.   Patients in relapse should be strongly encouraged to monitor calorie intake (7). Patients working on maintenance may have taken a "break" from monitoring and found great relief in doing so. A practitioner's suggestion to start recording again may be met with reluctance on the part of some patients. In such cases, practitioners may emphasize that recording is not a "life sentence" but rather one of many strategies that can help get patients back on track. "Portion distortions" and a general decrease in awareness of intake can arise over time and lead to relapse. Self-monitoring is required to make sure daily calorie totals are in line with goals. It is also helpful for patients to record their weight daily.

Meal Replacements.   One of the most effective ways to simplify choice and to decrease calorie intake is to start a structured meal plan, using meal replacements (such as shakes) and/or portion-controlled meals. These will help patients to keep their calorie intake in check. Using meal replacements or any of the prepackaged frozen entrees has many advantages. Such meals save the patient time (patients do not have to spend any time thinking about what to prepare for a meal or preparing it), reduce exposure to foods that might tempt patients to overeat, and avoid problems of underestimating portion sizes.

Structured Meal Plans. Another way to increase structure in the diet is to provide patients with a short-term, low-calorie, low-fat meal plan. Such short-term plans simplify food choices and increase adherence to a daily calorie goal. Patients need to weigh and measure foods to ensure appropriate portion sizes. This short-term structure can help give a new start and break the pattern of relapse.

Self-Selected Diet. A final dietary option is to have patients select foods of their choosing and calculate their cost in calorie and fat gram counters. This requires patients to weigh and measure their foods. When using this strategy, it is important for patients to be diligent about looking up foods throughout the day, so that they will know how close they are to reaching their calorie target.

Pharmacological Intervention

Patients who have lost weight via pharmacotherapy will likely benefit from continued use. Patients who have difficulty reversing small weight gains using the standard behavioral techniques described above may benefit from integrating pharmacotherapy into their program. Currently, sibutramine and orlistat are approved for use in the treatment of obesity in patients with a body mass index (BMI) $\geq$ 30 or in patients with a BMI $\geq$ 27 who have one or more obesity-related risk factors (eg, hypertension or dyslipidemia) (8,9). Patients for whom these medications are appropriate should be seen by a physician frequently, to monitor the medication and its potential side effects (see Chapter 7: Pharmacological Treatment).

Medication is most effective for maintenance when combined with a comprehensive program of behavior modification that includes frequent patient-provider contact (10,11). It is important to communicate to patients that medication is not a "magic bullet." The medication may make it easier to adhere to a low-calorie, low-fat diet, but it also requires significant effort on the part of the patient to eat less, exercise more, and maintain healthful behavior changes.

Strategies to Enhance Patient Motivation

Patients who are experiencing a decline in motivation may feel like they have given up some of the positive aspects of eating and leading a sedentary lifestyle and have likely become increasingly aware of the negative aspects of weight maintenance. They will often report being "sick of" the effort it takes to remain physically active and/or bored with trying to select healthy foods.

When the negative aspects of maintaining weight loss outweigh the positives, patients may become unmotivated and may begin to regain their weight. For example, JoAnne's weight has increased for the sixth week in a row, and she is inching closer to her baseline weight. She seems to have lost motivation. What can be done? The challenge for the practitioner is to find new ways to help patients stay motivated to maintain their healthful habits. Some suggestions are provided here.

Making a List of Positive Changes

Setting future goals is important. Patients focus on what they have not yet done or on how much weight they would eventually like to lose, rather than on what they have achieved. In such cases, it may be helpful for patients to make a list of the positive changes they have made that have enabled them to lose and maintain their weight loss. Practitioners may ask patients to recall what eating and exercise was like before they began losing weight. What are they doing differently now? Do they exercise more frequently? Wear different-size clothing? Walk stairs without getting winded? Realizing accomplishments may help increase motivation by increasing awareness of the positive changes.

Renewing Reasons for Maintaining Weight

Individuals may also find it helpful to make a list of the reasons why they would like to maintain weight loss. What benefits will occur in terms of their health, looks, or mood if they maintain their habit changes? Some patients may find that looking at a picture of themselves at their lowest weight helps trigger the benefits of maintaining their lower weight. Patients may also compare lab tests and/or blood pressure readings before weight loss and now.

Making the Negative Aspects of Weight-Loss Maintenance Less Negative

What is making it particularly difficult for the patient to maintain a healthy eating and exercise regimen? What aspects of weight maintenance are the most bothersome? What is getting in the way? Practitioners can help the patient explore ways to make the bothersome things less so. For example, if patients report that they are bored with the foods they are eating, buying a new low-fat cookbook or subscribing to a healthy cooking magazine could help. If they are tired of walking on the treadmill, maybe they could move their workout outdoors, try a new activity, or listen to a book on tape while they walk. Suggest at least one change the patient could make to reduce the troublesome aspects of weight maintenance.

Setting Goals and Rewards

Setting goals, both large and small, and rewards may be the best means of increasing motivation. Help patients select a long-term, challenging goal, such as completing a 5K race or raising money for a charity walk. However, smaller goals that can be achieved right away should also be identified. For example, the patient could call a friend to set up an exercise date for tomorrow, dispose of the high-calorie foods at home, or pack a healthy salad to bring to work.

Incentives that are tied to goals should be commensurate with the goals achieved. For short-term goals, patients may want to treat themselves to a massage or a manicure, purchase a new book or magazine, or go to a movie. Health-promoting rewards may also be used (see Box 9B.1). For larger goals, one option is to have patients put a dollar in a box every day the goal is met. At the end of the month, the patient can buy something with the money.

Finding a Partner

Just having company can sometimes be an effective motivator. Patients often report that time passes quickly when exercising with a friend. In addition, patients are likely to stay motivated to continue exercising if they know someone is waiting for them to exercise. Patients can be encouraged to find support by seeking out others interested in exercise and weight control by joining weight-loss meetings, biking clubs, aerobic classes, or a gym.

Box 9B.1. Examples of Health-Promoting Rewards for Achieving Goals

New exercise attire
A healthy cookbook
A quality nonstick skillet
Books on tape or music to listen to while walking
Registration for a physical activity class (eg, sports or a dance class)
Registration for a low-fat, low-calorie cooking class
Tickets for zoos and museums

Box 9B.2. For the Clinician: Handling Burnout

Practitioners working with patients who are regaining weight may become frustrated or even burned out. Being aware of how frustration could interfere with compassionate care is the first step in coping. Consulting with other practitioners for ways to help the patient (and practitioner) change course is often the best resource. It may be helpful to identify ways to "spice up" the intervention, such as a field trip to investigate the patient's cupboards at home, food shopping together, or a change in treatment modalities (eg, from individual to group treatment). Introducing other providers to the treatment, such as exercise physiologists, nutritionists, psychologists, or even chefs and wardrobe consultants, can also be helpful. Patients who are regaining weight during a prolonged period of time (eg, 6 months or more), despite the practitioner's best efforts, should consider delaying further weight control treatment until the timing improves. Ultimately, instead of feeling frustrated and hopeless, the practitioner should accept that the patient is having trouble and should be sympathetic during these difficult times.

Final Note

Successful weight maintenance is achievable but requires a consistent effort and diligence at exercising and consuming a low-calorie, low-fat diet. Maintenance may be improved by maximizing contact with participants, including high levels of exercise within treatment, providing structured approaches to dietary intake, and enhancing problem-solving skills. Moreover, revisiting patients' reasons for weight control, setting specific goals and rewards, and increasing social support may help patients stay motivated to maintain their healthy habits long-term.

References

1. Perri MG, Shapiro RM, Ludwig WW, Twentyman CT, McAdoo WG. Maintenance strategies for the treatment of obesity: an evaluation of relapse prevention training and post-treatment contact by telephone and mail. *J Consult Clin Psychol*. 1984;52:404–413.
2. Klem ML, Wing RR, McGuire MT, Seagle HM, Hill JO. A descriptive study of individuals successful at long-term maintenance of substantial weight loss. *Am J Clin Nutr*. 1997;66:239–246.
3. Lichtman SW, Pisarska K, Berman ER, Pestone M, Dowling H, Offenbacher E, Weisel H, Heshka S, Matthews DE, Heymsfield SB. Discrepancy between self-reported and actual caloric intake and exercise in obese subjects. *N Engl J Med*. 1992;327:1893–1898.

4. Perri MG, Nezu AM, McKelvey WF, Shermer RL, Renjilian DA, Viegener BJ. Relapse prevention training and problem-solving therapy in the long-term management of obesity. *J Consult Clin Psychol.* 2001;69:722–726.
5. Grilo CM, Shiffman S, Wing RR. Relapse crises and coping among dieters. *J Consult Clin Psychol.* 1989;57:488–495.
6. McGuire MT, Wing RR, Klem ML, Lang W, Hill JO. What predicts weight regain in a group of successful weight losers? *J Consult Clin Psychol.* 1999;67: 177–185.
7. Boutelle KN, Kirschenbaum DS. Further support for consistent self-monitoring as a vital component of successful weight control. *Obes Res.* 1998;6:219–224.
8. National Institutes of Health. Clinical guidelines on the identification, evaluation, and treatment of overweight and obesity in adults—the evidence report. *Obes Res.* 1998;6(Suppl 2):51S–209S.
9. National Task Force on the Prevention and Treatment of Obesity. Long-term pharmacotherapy in the management of obesity. *JAMA.* 1996;276:1907–1915.
10. Davidson MH, Hauptman J, DiGirolamo M, Foreyt JP, Halsted CH, Heber D, Heimburger DC, Lucas CP, Robbins DC, Chung J, Heymsfield SB. Weight control and risk factor reduction in obese subjects treated for 2 years with orlistat: a randomized controlled trial. *JAMA.* 1999;281:235–242.
11. James WP, Astrup A, Finer N, Hilsted J, Kopelman P, Rossner S, Saris WH, Van Gaal LF. Effect of sibutramine on weight maintenance after weight loss: a randomised trial. STORM Study Group. Sibutramine Trial of Obesity Reduction and Maintenance. *Lancet.* 2000;356:2119–2125.

Chapter 10
Patient and Professional Resources

Betty Kovacs, MS, RD

The nature of clinical visits has changed over the years as avenues for communicating have broadened. It is often not enough to hand a patient written information; to be thorough, it is important to also identify other resources the individual can use: Web sites, journals, newsletters, exercise videos, etc. The following resources are meant to be a resource for the practitioner and patient alike. This list is meant to give the reader a good foundation from which to find responsible information. Although it is by no means exhaustive, the list is a good representation of what is available, with particular emphasis on resources that are scientifically based.

Nutrition and Health Resources

General Information and Research Web Sites

Food and Nutrition Information Center (FNIC)
http://www.nal.usda.gov/fnic

One of several information centers located at the National Agricultural Library (NAL), Agricultural Research Service (ARS), US Department of Agriculture (USDA). Contains more than 1,800 links to current and reliable nutrition information.

Healthfinder
http://www.healthfinder.gov
    A free guide to reliable health information, developed by the US Department of Health and Human Services. Provides an easy-to-use, searchable index of carefully reviewed health information from more than 1,800 government agencies, nonprofit organizations, and universities.

Healthy People 2010
http://www.healthypeople.gov
    Healthy People 2010 is the prevention agenda for the United States. It is a statement of national health objectives designed to identify the most significant preventable threats to health and to establish national goals to reduce these threats.

HerbalWatch.com
http://www.herbalwatch.com
    Profiles the marketing of herbs, the bogus advertising of herbs, and the harmful effects of herbs.

Medscape
http://www.medscape.com
    Offers health professionals medical information and education tools. Key features include MEDLINE searches, conference coverage, a primary-source medical journal (*Medscape General Medicine*) and professional medical news from Reuters, Medscape Medical News, and medical news journal publishers.

National Center for Health Statistics
http://www.cdc.gov/nchs
    Includes an overview of the Centers for Disease Control and Prevention's major data collection activities and data-based findings. Provides information about special activities and initiatives to improve access to, and the quality of, health statistics information. Offers links to additional sources of health information and provides a way to query electronically to obtain answers to specific questions.

National Library of Medicine
http://www.nlm.nih.gov/medlineplus/obesity.html
    Provides information about nutrition and about treatment of obesity, as well as links to the latest news, recent research, and nutrition and clinical trials.

National Women's Health Information Center (NWHIC)
http://www.4women.org
    NWHIC is a service of the Office on Women's Health, in the Department of Health and Human Services. Provides a wide variety of women's health-related material, developed by the Department of Health and Human Services, other Federal agencies, and private-sector resources.

New York Online Access to Health (NOAH)
http://www.noah-health.org
Provides access to full-text consumer health information in English and Spanish.

National Heart, Lung, and Blood Institute (NHLBI)
Obesity Education Initiative
http://www.nhlbi.nih.gov/guidelines/obesity/ob_home.htm
The National Heart, Lung, and Blood Institute (NHLBI), of the National Institutes of Health (NIH), launched the Obesity Education Initiative (OEI) in January 1991. Its purpose is to help reduce the prevalence of overweight and physical inactivity, to reduce the risk of coronary heart disease.

Nutrition.gov
http://www.nutrition.gov
This new federal resource provides easy access to all on-line federal government information on nutrition, healthy eating, physical activity, and food safety.

NutriWatch
http://www.nutriwatch.com
NutriWatch provides comprehensive information about nutrition and food safety, including full-text copies or links to source documents that would be useful to educators, students, and journalists.

Partnership for Healthy Weight Management
http://www.consumer.gov/weightloss/
A coalition of representatives from science, academia, the health care profession, government, commercial enterprises, and organizations whose mission is to promote sound guidance on strategies for achieving and maintaining a healthy weight. The Partnership issues Voluntary Guidelines for Providers of Weight Loss Products or Services, to encourage weight-loss programs and to provide consumers with basic program information.

PubMed
http://www.ncbi.nih.gov/entrez/query.fcgi
Provides free access for users to perform MEDLINE searches. It was developed by the National Center for Biotechnology Information (NCBI) at the National Library of Medicine (NLM), located at the National Institutes of Health (NIH).

Tufts Nutrition Navigator
http://navigator.tufts.edu/
Designed to help individuals sort through the large volume of nutrition information on the Internet and to find accurate, useful nutrition information.

WebMD
http://www.webmd.com

A consumer-focused health care information Web site. Provides health and wellness news, support communities, interactive health management tools, and more. The site's on-line communities and special events allow consumers to participate in real-time discussions with experts and with other people who share similar health conditions or concerns.

Weight-control Information Network (WIN)
http://www.niddk.nih.gov/health/nutrit/win.htm

A national information service of the National Institute of Diabetes and Digestive and Kidney Diseases (NIDDK), National Institutes of Health (NIH). Established in 1994 to provide health professionals and consumers with science-based information on obesity, weight control, and nutrition, WIN provides publications (fact sheets, brochures, article reprints, and conference and workshop proceedings), videotaped lectures, and a quarterly newsletter.

Newsletters

American Institute for Cancer Research (AICR) Newsletter
http://www.aicr.org
800/843-8114

AICR's quarterly newsletter explains current cancer research, provides recipes and menu ideas for healthy eating, and offers practical advice to lower cancer risk.

Consumer Health Digest
http://www.ncahf.org/digest/chd.html

A free weekly e-mail newsletter edited by Stephen Barrett, MD, and cosponsored by NCAHF and Quackwatch. It summarizes scientific reports, legislative developments, enforcement actions, other news items, Web site evaluations, recommended and nonrecommended books, research tips, and other information relevant to consumer protection and consumer decision-making.

Consumer Reports on Health
http://www.consumerreports.org
800/333-9784

A 12-page, monthly newsletter based on expert advice from leading medical authorities from the United States and around the world.

Environmental Nutrition
http://www.environmentalnutrition.com
800/829-5384

Monthly newsletter that provides sensible, practical guidance on foods that will, for instance, help lower the risk of heart disease, cancer, or diabetes.

FDA Consumer
http://www.fda.gov/fdac/
888/INFO-FDA
The official magazine of the Food and Drug Administration (FDA). *FDA Consumer* is bimonthly and offers in-depth information on how to get healthy and stay healthy. It also reports on current FDA activities, to ensure that the products the agency regulates—food, human and animal drugs, medical devices, cosmetics, radiation-emitting products, and biologics—are fit to use.

Harvard Health Publications
http://www.health.harvard.edu
Harvard Medical School produces five monthly newsletters: *Harvard Health Letter, Harvard Mental Health Letter, Harvard Heart Letter, Harvard Women's Health Watch,* and *Harvard Men's Health Watch*.

Health Facts and Fears
http://www.healthfactsandfears.com
The webzine of the American Council on Science and Health, which strives to separate real health risks from media and activist scare stories.

Mayo Clinic Health Letter
http://www.mayohealth.org
800/333-9037
An 8-page, monthly newsletter on health and medical news. Articles draw on the expertise of more than 1,100 Mayo Clinic physicians.

Nutrition Action Health Letter
http://www.cspinet.org
202/332-9110
The Center for Science in the Public Interest (CSPI) is a nonprofit education and advocacy organization that focuses on improving the safety and nutritional quality of our food supply and on reducing the carnage caused by alcoholic beverages. *Nutrition Action Health Letter* publishes ten issues per calendar year.

Tufts University Health & Nutrition Letter
http://www.healthletter.tufts.edu
800/274-7581
Provides scientific-based information on health. Offers advice on choosing food wisely, controlling weight, preventing disease, and staying fit.

UC Berkeley Wellness Letter
http://www.berkeleywellness.com
386/447-6328

This well-researched monthly newsletter reviews the latest research and clarifies the often conflicting and superficial health information presented by the popular media.

Professional Journals

Obesity Research
http://www.obesityresearch.org/

The official journal of the North American Association for the Study of Obesity (NAASO). Covers the latest research about obesity.

International Journal of Obesity
http://www.nature.com/ijo

Contains articles about obesity and its relationship to biochemistry, physiology, genetics, nutrition, metabolism, psychology, behavior, and epidemiology.

Obesity Reviews
http://www.blackwell-synergy.com

Official journal of the International Association for the Study of Obesity. Publishes updated reviews in all disciplines related to obesity.

Obesity Surgery
http://www.obesitysurgery.com

Official journal of the American Society of Bariatric Surgeons. Contains the latest research on surgical techniques and outcomes.

Weight-Management Programs

eDiets
http://www.ediets.com
800/987-6824

The largest subscription-based on-line diet, fitness, and counseling network. The customized diet programs are based on individual members' personal goals, food preferences, and lifestyles. In addition, eDiets.com publishes a biweekly diet and fitness e-mail newsletter.

Dietwatch
http://www.dietwatch.com

Provides individuals who are interested in fitness, weight loss, and health the tools, supportive community, and information they need to reach a healthy weight and lifestyle. Also provides an active community, available for individuals who support each other in their efforts to reach a healthful weight and lifestyle.

Nutrawatch
http://www.nutrawatch.com

Designed to help individuals track the nutritional content of foods. This is useful for those following a special diet for physical fitness training for medical reasons, or for weight loss. A database of foods enables users to quickly find and record what they have eaten.

Overeaters Anonymous (OA)
http://www.overeatersanonymous.org
World Service Office: 505/891-2664

Offers support groups based on a 12-step program. OA charges no dues or fees; it is self-supporting through member contributions. It is not a religious organization and does not promote any particular diet. To address weight loss, OA encourages members to develop a food plan with a health care professional and a sponsor.

PACE (Patient-centered Assessment & Counseling for Exercise & Nutrition)
http://www.paceproject.org

PACE is a comprehensive approach to brief physical activity and nutrition counseling using materials developed by a team of researchers at San Diego State University.

Shape Up America!
http://www.shapeup.org

A national initiative to promote healthy weight and increased physical activity in the United States. Involves a broad-based coalition of industry, medical/health, nutrition, physical fitness, and related organizations and experts.

TOPS (Take off Pounds Sensibly)
http://www.tops.org
518/438-8928

Started in 1948, TOPS now has support groups in every state and in 20 countries. TOPS endorses the American Dietetic Association exchange program but will not recommend any specific diet without physician approval. Members attend group sessions that provide information, motivation, and fellowship, to help them attain their weight-loss goal.

Weight Watchers International, Inc.
http://www.weightwatchers.com
800/651-6000

One of the most accepted, nonphysician supervised, weight-management programs in the world. Their diet plan is high in fiber, fruits, and vegetables, and it follows government guidelines. Groups are taught by successful Weight Watchers participants. They also offer on-line support for those unable or unwilling to go to meetings. Weight Watchers food is available in supermarkets but is not sold on-line.

Sources of Meal Replacements and Low-Calorie Diets

HMR
http://www.hmrprogram.com
Consumer information: 800/418-1367

This weight-management program is franchised by medical centers across the country and the program is physician supervised. The program contains modules combining information on behavior, nutrition, and activity. Groups are taught by health professionals. A very-low-calorie diet program that offers a combination of liquid- and regular-food meal replacements.

Jenny Craig Inc.
http://www.jennycraig.com
800/775-JENNY

A commercial weight-loss program in Jenny Craig Centers. Weight loss is supervised by employees trained by the company. Food guidelines are given, but Jenny Craig meals are also purchased by participants.

Optifast
http://www.optifast.com

Part of Sandoz Pharmaceuticals, this very-low-calorie-diet program is also franchised by medical centers across the country, and the program is physician supervised. Contains modules combining information on behavior, nutrition, and activity. Groups are taught by health professionals. A combination of liquid and food bars is prescribed.

SlimFast
http://www.slimfast.com

A free on-line community that provides such features as an on-line buddy program, weight chart, food diary, and hundreds of free recipes. There is information from registered dietitians, exercise physiologists, and professional chefs.

Food Facts

All Recipes
http://www.allrecipes.com
206/292-3990

American Academy of Family Physicians
http://familydoctor.org/cgi-bin/list.pl?element=handout

American Dietetic Association
Nutrition Fact Sheets
http://www.eatright.org

American Egg Board
http://www.aeb.org
847/296-7043

Cooking Light
http://www.cookinglight.com

Cooking Measures and Conversion Calculator
http://www.globalgourmet.com/cgi-bin/hts?convcalc.hts+oven+new

Food and Health Communications
http://www.foodandhealth.com/handout.shtml

Food Guide Pyramid
http://www.nal.usda.gov/fnic/Fpyr/pyramid.html

National Dairy Council
http://www.nationaldairycouncil.org

Nutrient Data Laboratory
http://www.nal.usda.gov/fnic/foodcomp

Produce for Better Health Foundation
http://www.5aday.com
302/235-2329

The Vegetarian Resource Group
http://www.vrg.org
410/366-VEGE

Wheat Foods Council
http://www.wheatfoods.org
303/840-8787

Physical Activity Resources

Pamphlet

Active at Any Size
http://www.niddk.nih.gov/health/nutrit/activeatanysize/active.html

Advice for very large individuals who want to become more active. Available from the National Institutes of Diabetes and Digestive and Kidney Diseases (Bethesda, Md: National Institutes of Health; 2001. NIH Publication No. 00-4352).

Videos

Chair Dancing
http://www.chairdancing.com
800/551-4386
    No-impact video series designed to improve muscle tone, flexibility, and cardiovascular endurance without putting stress on your knees, back, hips, or feet.

Step Counter Distributors

New Lifestyles
http://www.new-lifestyles.com
888/748-5377

Accusplit
http://www.accusplit.com
800/935-1996

Internet Resource

Healthy Living with Bliss
http://www.KellyBliss.com
    Information on fitness activities for large and very large people. A resource section includes fitness wear, books, exercise equipment, classes, and information on where to buy fitness videos for large people.

Medical Resources

Clinical Trials and Research

Center Watch
http://www.centerwatch.com
    Provides an extensive list of Internal Review Board–approved clinical trials being conducted internationally, many of which are open for public participation. Also lists promising therapies newly approved by the FDA.

Look Ahead Study
http://www.lookaheadstudy.org

Sponsored by the National Institutes of Health, this is the first clinical research to look at the long-term health effects of weight loss in men and women who are overweight and have type 2 diabetes. About 5,000 people, ages 45 to 75 years, who have type 2 diabetes will participate in 16 centers nationwide. They know that weight loss has many short-term benefits, but they don't know whether these benefits last for many years. This project will help us to understand the long-term effects of weight loss on health, especially on heart attack and stroke.

The National Weight Control Registry (NWCR)
http://www.lifespan.org/services/bmed/wt_loss/nwcr/
800/606-NWCR

NWCR is a research study that has exploded the myth that everyone who loses weight gains it back. It has shown that successful weight loss is indeed possible. Nearly 3,000 individuals have been identified who have lost significant amounts of weight and have kept it off for long periods of time. Recruitment for the registry is ongoing. If an individual is at least 18 years of age and has maintained at least a 30-lb weight loss for 1 year or longer, he or she may be eligible to join the research study.

Health Misinformation and Fraud

American Council on Science and Health (ACSH)
http://www.acsh.org
212/362-7044

Presents balanced, scientifically sound analyses of current health topics. ACSH is a unique voice, backed by mainstream science, defending the achievements and benefits of responsible technology within America's free-enterprise system.

Consumer Lab
http://www.consumerlab.com
914/722-9149

Provides independent test results and information to help consumers and health care professionals evaluate health, wellness, and nutrition products. It publishes results of its tests on-line, including listings of brands that have passed testing.

Federal Trade Commission
http://www.ftc.gov/bcp/menu-health.htm

Information on deceptive diet advertisements and how to tell the realistic programs from the unrealistic.

National Council Against Health Fraud
http://www.ncahf.org
978/532-9383
A private, nonprofit, voluntary health agency that focuses on health misinformation, fraud, and quackery as public health problems. Their positions are based on the principles of science that underlie consumer protection law.

Quackwatch
http://www.quackwatch.org
Quackwatch, Inc., a member of Consumer Federation of America, is a nonprofit corporation whose purpose is to combat health-related frauds, myths, fads, and fallacies. Its primary focus is on quackery-related information that is difficult or impossible to get elsewhere.

Sources of FDA-Approved Medications

Abbott Laboratories
http://4meridia.com
800/633-9110
Producer of sibutramine (Meridia).

Hoffmann-La Roche Inc
973/235-5000
http://www.xenical.com
http://www.xenicare.com
Producer of orlistat (Xenical)

Psychology and Behavior Resources

Eating Disorder Referral and Information Center
http://www.edreferral.com
Provides information and treatment resources for all forms of eating disorders. The center's goal is to provide assistance, in the form of information and resources, to those with eating disorders, to get them started on the road to recovery and healthy living.

National Eating Disorders Association
http://www.nationaleatingdisorders.org
206/382-3587
The largest nonprofit organization in the United States dedicated to the elimination of eating disorders and body dissatisfaction. They have developed prevention programs for a wide range of audiences, they publish and distribute educational materials, they operate the nation's first toll-free eat-

ing disorders information and referral line, and they continually work to change the cultural, familial, and interpersonal factors that contribute to the development of eating disorders and body dissatisfaction.

National Institute of Mental Health
http://www.nimh.nih.gov
301/443-4513

This is the sister site to the National Institutes of Health. Information for the public is clear and easily understood. Provides references and information for professionals, including clinical trials.

Body Image
http://www.body-images.com

Developed by Thomas Cash, PhD, a pioneer in the study of body image. Contains a variety of assessment tools and treatment materials related to body image.

Size Acceptance and Weight Discrimination Resources

Council on Weight Discrimination
http://www.cswd.org
845/679-1209

A not-for-profit advocacy organization working to end discrimination against people who are heavier than average.

Fat Friendly Health Professionals List
http://www.cat-and-dragon.com/stef/fat/ffp.html

A list of health professionals who have been deemed "fat friendly" or who have declared themselves "fat friendly," as well as other Web sites listing "fat friendly" health professionals. The list is arranged alphabetically by country, state, and city.

Grand Style
http://www.grandstyle.com

Size 14+ women can speak with experts, shop, learn more about fitness and entertaining, and locate hard-to-find products and services.

Largely Positive
http://www.largelypositive.com

Aims to teach people that their weight is not a measure of their self-worth and to give them tips on how to improve their self-image and self-esteem, even though they may occupy a larger body. The site is also educational in nature, dedicated to separating fact from fiction and to correcting the wealth of misinformation that exists about issues of size and weight.

Largesse
http://www.eskimo.com/~largesse
Largesse, the Network for Size Esteem, is an internationally recognized resource center and clearinghouse for size diversity empowerment.

National Association to Advance Fat Acceptance
http://www.naafa.org
916/558-6880
Seeks to end discrimination based on body size and to improve the quality of life for large people. It offers a variety of publications and videos on size acceptance, self-esteem, and health and fitness.

Size Wise
http://www.sizewise.com
Provides information and resources designed to make life healthier, more comfortable, and more enjoyable for heavier individuals.

Professional Associations

American Association of Diabetes Educators
http://www.aadenet.org
800/338-3633

American Cancer Society
http://www.cancer.org
800/ACS-2345

American College of Sports Medicine
http://www.acsm.org

American Diabetes Association
http://www.diabetes.org
800/DIABETES

American Dietetic Association
http://www.eatright.org
800/877-1600

American Heart Association
http://www.americanheart.org
800/AHA-USA-1

American Medical Association
http://www.ama-assn.org
312/464-5000

American Obesity Association
http://www.obesity.org
202/776-7711

American Sleep Apnea Association
http://www.sleepapnea.org
202/293-3650

American Society for Nutritional Sciences
http://www.asns.org
301/530-7050

American Society for Bariatric Surgery
http://www.asbs.org
352/331-4900

American Stroke Association
http://www.strokeassociation.org
888/4-STROKE

Diabetes Exercise and Sports Association
http://www.diabetes-exercise.org
800/808-4322

International Association for the Study of Obesity
http://www.iaso.org

National Association to Advance Fat Acceptance
http://www.naafa.org
916/558-6880

North American Association for the Study of Obesity (NAASO)
http://www.naaso.org
301/563-6526

Society for Nutrition Education
http://www.sne.org
800/235-6690

Sports, Cardiovascular and Wellness Nutritionists
http://www.scandpg.org
719/395-9271